The little Goddess book of big beauty ideas

Elisabeth Wilson

Acknowledgements
Infinite ideas would like to thank the following authors for their contributions to this book: Linda Bird, Sally Brown, Eve Cameron, Kate Cook, Cherry Maslen and Elisabeth Wilson.

First published in 2009 by
The Infinite Ideas Company Limited
36 St Giles
Oxford, OX1 3LD
United Kingdom
www.infideas.com

A CIP catalogue record for this book is available from the British Library

ISBN: 978-1-905940-88-2

Designed and typeset by Baseline Arts Ltd, Oxford
Printed in China

Lincolnshire
COUNTY COUNCIL
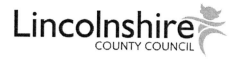

COMMUNITIES, CULTURAL SERVICES
and ADULT EDUCATION

This book should be returned on or before
the last date shown below.

NE4

GRANTHAM
581
16-12-10

To renew or order library books please telephone 01522 782010
or visit www.lincolnshire.gov.uk

You will require a Personal Identification Number.
Ask any member of staff for this.

Brilliant ideas

I want to be thin!

Look gorgeous every single day

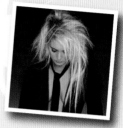

'Life is not about finding yourself, it's about creating yourself,' said George Bernard Shaw, and nowhere is this truer than when it comes to our appearance. It's relatively easy to transform the way we look – easier than changing our inner selves, for sure. And the great thing is that looking good does wonders for how we feel inside. Which is a virtuous circle as the secret to looking good is feeling confident. Whether you want smooth thighs, a flatter tummy or just some handy beauty quick-fixes this little book should have all the ideas you need to keep you looking your best 100% of the time.

'I don't want to make money.
I just want to be wonderful'
MARILYN MONROE

The beauty basics

Are you preventing yourself from being gorgeous?

You feel less than gorgeous. Could it be you that's the problem?

1. Where is your latest gas bill?
❑ Paid and filed (score 0)
❑ In the bottom of your handbag (1)
❑ You're not sure (2)

2. You're meeting some friends at the weekend.
❑ You're meeting at 7.30 on Saturday (score 0)
❑ You know it's Saturday but you'll set a time by texting in the afternoon (1)
❑ You're not sure you're going to make Saturday – you've double booked (2)

3. A friend has blagged an entrance to a starry film premiere. She can take you with her – but it's this evening. Do you...
❑ Rush home to slip into your favourite outfit, pressed and ready to wear (score 0)
❑ Manage to rustle together something but don't have the right tights or handbag at short notice (1)
❑ Buy a new outfit because you have no idea if you have anything suitable (2)

How did you do?

Score 3 or more and there's every chance you're not organised enough to be gorgeous. It takes application, it takes time and you're too busy looking for your mobile phone to get gorgeous.

4. The weekend, for you, is an opportunity to:
☐ Look gorgeous in cashmere and jeans (0)
☐ Get away with not wearing make-up (1)
☐ Get away with not washing (2)

5. You have been planning to lose 10lbs:
☐ And you will in time for summer/Christmas/John and Julie's wedding (0)
☐ It would be a lot easier if you could be bothered to exercise (1)
☐ And that's what it's likely to stay – a plan (2)

6. Your hair is cut
☐ Every six weeks (0)
☐ Every six months (1)
☐ When you can't see (2)

What does this mean?

Score 3 or more and you are too lazy to be gorgeous – we repeat, it takes application, it takes time. Your insouciance is admirable, just be careful it doesn't slip into total slobdom and if you'd like to be a little more appearance-orientated turn to idea 1, Boost your body image, to learn the basics of planning.

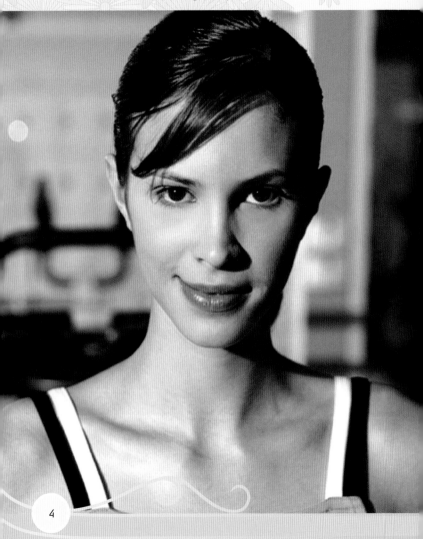

4

1. Boost your body image

Newsflash! You don't have to be beautiful to be perceived as such. The secret to looking good is feeling confident. Start with a few self-esteem tricks.

Take a minute to scroll through your list of female friends, colleagues and acquaintances. Not all lookers are they? Yet how many of those who aren't conventionally 'beautiful' exude a goddess-like aura nevertheless?

This is more than 'charm' and less obvious than raw sex appeal, although they may have that too. It's an intrinsic self-belief and *joie de vivre* that makes even 'homely' women somehow magnetic. Some people have bags of it. It may be something they were lucky enough to acquire in childhood. However, if *you* didn't acquire it, you don't need hours of therapy to get some too. Self-confidence (real or faked) is a beauty trick we can all learn.

Life coaches and shrinks suggest we tell ourselves at every opportunity how fantastic we are. In truth, most of us cringe at the thought, so I suggest listing your hottest qualities instead. Go on. Get a piece of paper and list them under a heading such as 'Things I Like About Myself' or 'My Best Bits'. See, I bet you feel better already. An alternative is to make a list of all the compliments you've received, from sweet nothings whispered by exes to ego-boosters that other women have bestowed upon you (which, bizarrely, often count for more). In moments of self-doubt, consult your list.

Here's an idea for you...

Fill a photo album with pictures in which you're looking your best and reach for it whenever low self-confidence is a problem.

Second, start focusing on and pampering the bits you love about yourself. So, if you've been told you have great legs, then capitalise on that. For example, indulge in some amazingly expensive body oil for them, buy yourself some unspeakably impractical shoes or add a few new leg-revealing mini skirts or floaty numbers to your wardrobe. And if your hair is your unique selling point, then get a haircut regularly and experiment with different looks or accessories. The key to recognising and accepting that you're attractive is to do all you can to glory in your best assets and show them off to their best advantage.

Pampering yourself on a regular basis is a great way to boost your self-confidence. How much more attractive do you feel after a facial/manicure or even after a spritz of a new perfume? It's not about spending a fortune, it's about recognising that pampery girly treats can really boost your *amour propre* and help you to ooze gorgeousness, even if it's simply taking a luxurious, gorgeous-smelling bath, or wearing your sexiest, most expensive clothes just for the hell of it. Start taking pleasure in looking your best.

But what if you're overweight/out of shape/flabbier than you were two, five or ten years ago and your wardrobe is testament to the nubile beauty you once were and not the gallumping great oaf you now are and are evermore destined to be? Well, you have two options here. First, do all the above. Second, throw out all those thin clothes (they'll only depress you) and start building up a completely new wardrobe of clothes that fit and flatter you.

I'd suggest that you start doing some exercise as well. Nothing excessive, just something gentle but regular. Simply moving your body can help boost your mood, improve your complexion and give you confidence in your shape. And before you know it you'll have lost pounds! Aim for about twenty minutes of exercise three times a week. It's quite addictive so you'll probably want to do more, but if you start to see it as a chore remind yourself that you're doing something positive to make the best of your shape and regard it as a short cut to self-belief instead. And how much cheaper is that than a facelift?

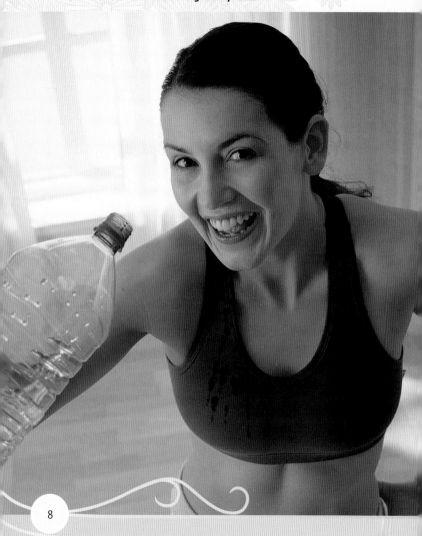

2. Water works

Water is a beauty tonic on tap. Eight glasses a day can boost your energy and make you slimmer, cleverer and more positive. Here's why.

GPs, nutritionists, dermatologists and beauty therapists all agree that drinking water is one surefire way to a longer, healthier life and plumper, firmer skin.

Water is involved in nearly every bodily function, from circulation to body temperature and from digestion to waste excretion. It helps your body to absorb the nutrients from food, too. When you get dehydrated, vitamins and minerals aren't absorbed optimally and toxins can't get excreted as efficiently. Food is like a sponge; if it's saturated with water it swells and allows the vitamins and minerals into your body, which can help heal you and boost your immune system. Water is also necessary for lubricating joints and providing a protective cushion for the body's many organs and tissues. And, when you're not getting enough water, your blood volume drops, which stops you from firing on all cylinders. All of this affects how you feel and how you look.

So, how much water do we really need? The Natural Mineral Water Information Service estimates that about 90% of us don't get enough fluids. This deficiency has been linked to headaches, lethargy, dry skin, digestive problems and even mood swings. Many medical bodies recommend that a 60 kg adult drinks 1.5 to 2 litres (between six and

Here's an idea for you...

You can eat your fluids, too. Fruit and vegetables are largely water – apricots, grapes, melons, peaches, strawberries, cucumbers, mangoes, oranges and peppers are all more than 75% water. Fish such as sardines, mackerel, salmon and tuna are also 50% water.

eight 250 ml glasses) of fluids a day, plenty of which should be water. Alternatively, aim for about 30 ml of water per kg of your body weight or 1 litre for every 1,000 calories of food you consume.

Your best gauge is the colour of your urine. You're after a pale watery colour with a tinge of lemon; yellow urine means you need to drink more.

If you're partying, match a glass of water for every alcoholic drink. And drink at least half a cup of water for each drink containing caffeine (such as tea, coffee or cola) to counteract their diuretic effect. Sipping is better than gulping huge glasses at a time. Experts say that the latter is just like pouring water on a dry leaf, so is certainly not the best way to absorb it.

Beauty booster: water can help you lose weight

How often do you confuse hunger with thirst and end up reaching for food instead of drinking? This is very common, but will cost you dearly in calories. Research shows that 75% of all hunger pangs are actually thirst, so if you get the munchies and fancy a Mars Bar, try a glass of water instead and save yourself some calories.

One study showed that you could increase your metabolic rate by about 30% by having a big 500 ml glass of cold water after each meal. This comes down to a process called thermogenesis, in other words the rate at which your body burns calories for digestion. Apparently, drinking cold water means you'll burn off your supper that much quicker! Another study found that drinking 2 litres of water daily can help your body to burn off an extra 150 calories a day. This can also flatten your tum because it can help you beat the water retention that causes bloated bellies.

Defining idea...

'Beauty of style and harmony and grace and good rhythm depend on simplicity.'
PLATO

Beauty booster: water can make you feel brighter and more energised

No one looks their best when they're exhausted. Drinking water has been found to refresh both physically and mentally so can enhance your performance. Studies show it helps concentration and assimilation of information, so if you swig regularly you'll feel brighter and radiate perkiness.

Beauty booster: water is great for your skin

Whenever you're dehydrated, your body effectively steals water from less important parts of your body and delivers it to the more important organs, so your skin is the first place it'll show if you're not drinking enough. Water can also help reduce puffy skin and eyes because it decreases the amount of salt in your body. Drink a glass before you go to bed and sleep on a thick pillow or with your head elevated to help prevent fluid from settling under your eyes.

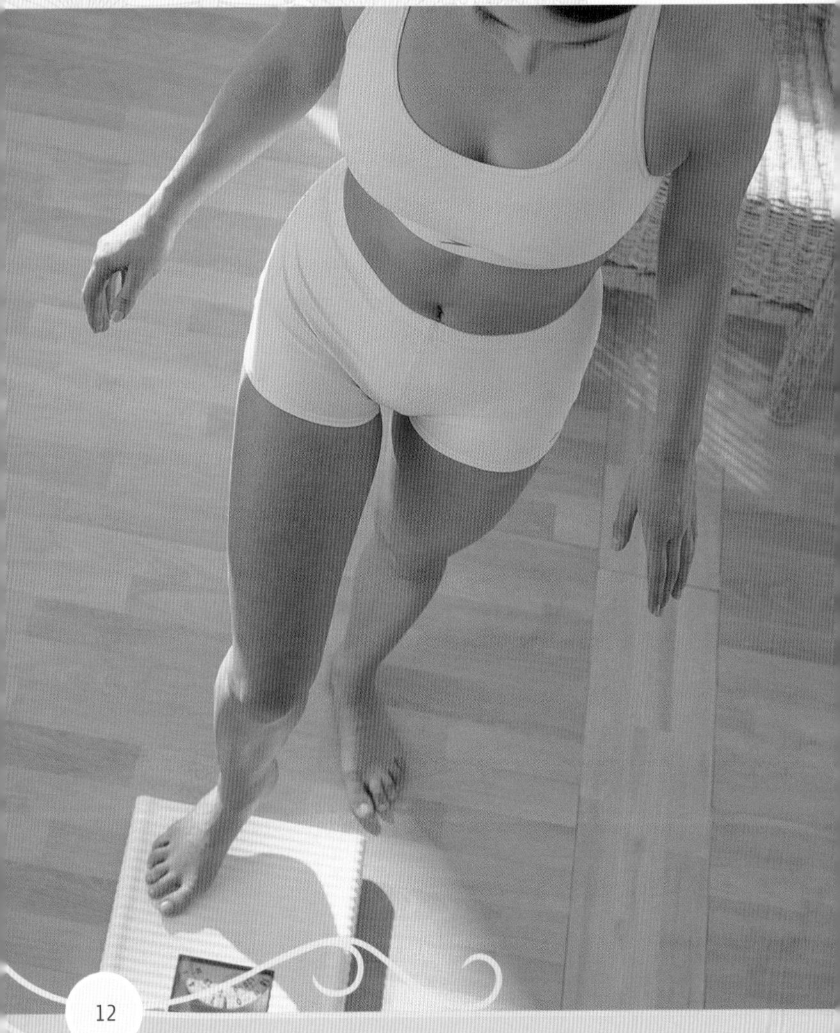

3. Lose pounds without trying

Kiss goodbye to diets. There are easier, less painful ways to lose weight – and keep it off. A few simple lifestyle changes may be all you need to drop a dress size.

The year I gave up dieting I lost more weight than I'd ever managed before. Still, diets are a kind of rite of passage. Every woman's tried one – and has usually ended up obsessed with food and calories.

When I worked at *Zest* magazine, the editorial policy was never to cover diets that you 'go on' and 'come off' again. We knew from personal experience that they didn't work and dozens of experts had confirmed exactly that. Instead, we talked in terms of eating habits: healthier choices and food for lifestyle.

Diets don't work because they're offering short-term solutions that are impossible to sustain in the long term. You either feel so hungry, deprived or bored that you instantly crave that which you're not allowed or your nutrition is so unbalanced that your body steers you towards the calories it craves.

So, here are ten golden rules of healthy eating that really will help you to shed pounds without suffering:

Here's an idea for you...

Simplify your diet: experts say that if you're presented with a large variety of foods you tend to eat more.

1 Don't skip breakfast

Skipping breakfast won't help you to save calories and lose pounds. On the contrary, when you do eat breakfast you're more likely to make better, lower-calorie choices throughout the rest of the day because it'll kick-start your metabolism and give you the whole day to burn calories. Also, your body is more efficient at processing carbohydrates in the morning.

2 Eat lots of fibre

A high-fibre diet is one of the best ways to lose weight. One study showed that people who ate a low-fat diet that included 26 g of fibre per 1,000 calories lost more weight than those whose diet was higher in fat and lower in fibre (just 7 g per day). That may sound a lot, but you can up your fibre intake by eating bran cereals, wholemeal pasta, wholemeal bread and lots of fruit and vegetables.

3 Eat little and often

The aim of this one is to maintain your blood sugar level at a level where you don't get really hungry and end up reaching for the biscuit tin. It will also keep your metabolism working efficiently all day. So, divide your calorie intake into five or six smaller meals or choose regular healthy snacks such as crackers, yoghurt, fruit and nuts.

4 Watch your portions

As a rough guide, a portion of carbohydrate (e.g. pasta, rice or potatoes) should fit into the palm of your hand. The same goes for protein (fish, meat, cheese, etc.). As for fruit and vegetables, you can eat your fill.

Defining idea...

'I feel about airplanes the way I feel about diets. It seems to me that they are wonderful things for other people to go on.'
JEAN KERR, writer

5 Control the booze

Booze is full of empty calories that can't be stored so the body uses them first and then stores as fat anything else you've eaten surplus to your body's requirements. Booze can also weaken your resolve so that a curry, for example, is likely to become much more appealing after a few beers. Keep track of your tipples so that you don't exceed your daily alcohol allowance.

6 Eat more slowly

If you gobble your food you'll end up eating more. It takes about twenty minutes for your brain and stomach to compute that you're full up, so make mealtimes more leisurely. Always sit down to eat, put your fork down between bites and chew your food thoroughly before you swallow.

Defining idea...

'The only way to lose fat is to take in fewer calories than your body needs. It's as simple as that.'
ANITA BEAN, nutritionist

7 Be supermarket savvy

Never shop hungry and always make a list so that you're less likely to succumb to those tasty but high-fat 'two for one' offers or the crisps and chocolate at the checkout. And unless you're doing a big weekly shop, always use a basket rather than a trolley so that by the time you've bought your essentials, you can't carry anything else!

8 Use smaller plates

Swap those whopping dinner plates for smaller ones about 20 cm in diameter (a dinner plate is usually about 25 to 30 cm in diameter), as people tend to clear their plates regardless of how many calories this means they eat.

9 Go easy on evening carbs

You're unlikely to use many carbs after dinner so they'll probably be stored as fat. Instead, eat protein, such as fish, and lots of vegetables.

10 Eat fruit or salad before meals

One study showed that women who ate a little apple or pear before each meal lost more weight than women who skipped the fruit but followed the same reduced-calorie diet. Fruit is full of fibre, so it can help fill you up. In another study, people who ate a low-fat 100-calorie salad before their meal ate about 12% less than those who didn't have the salad.

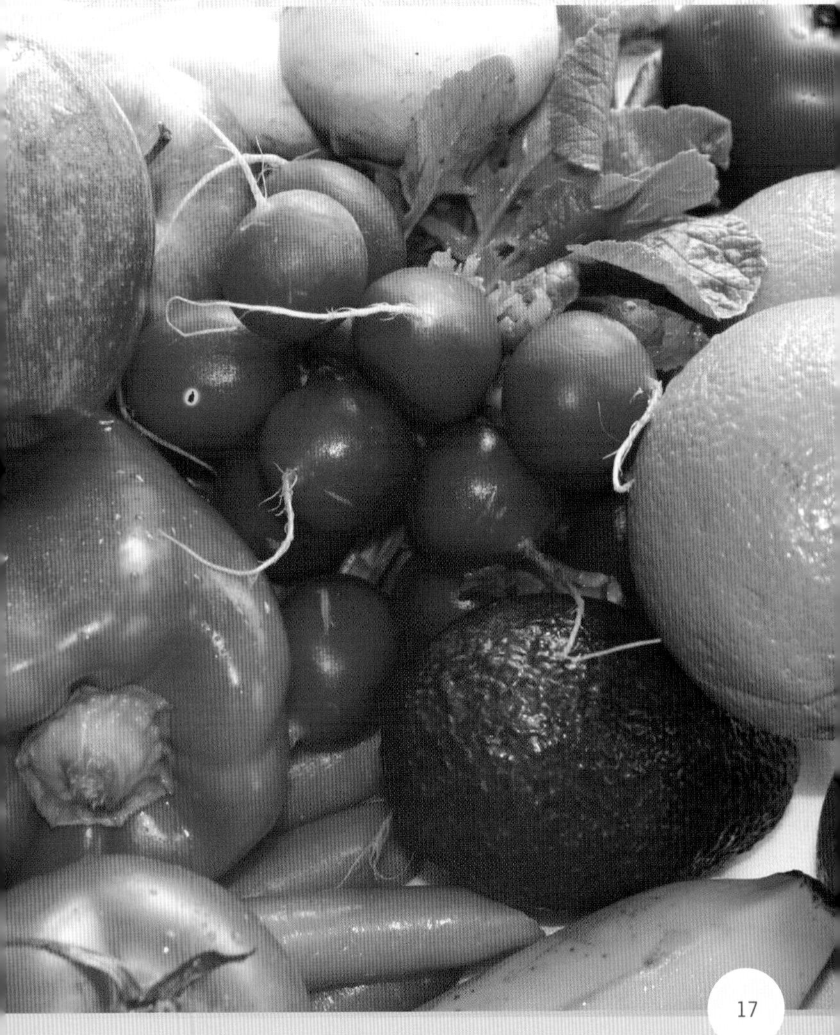

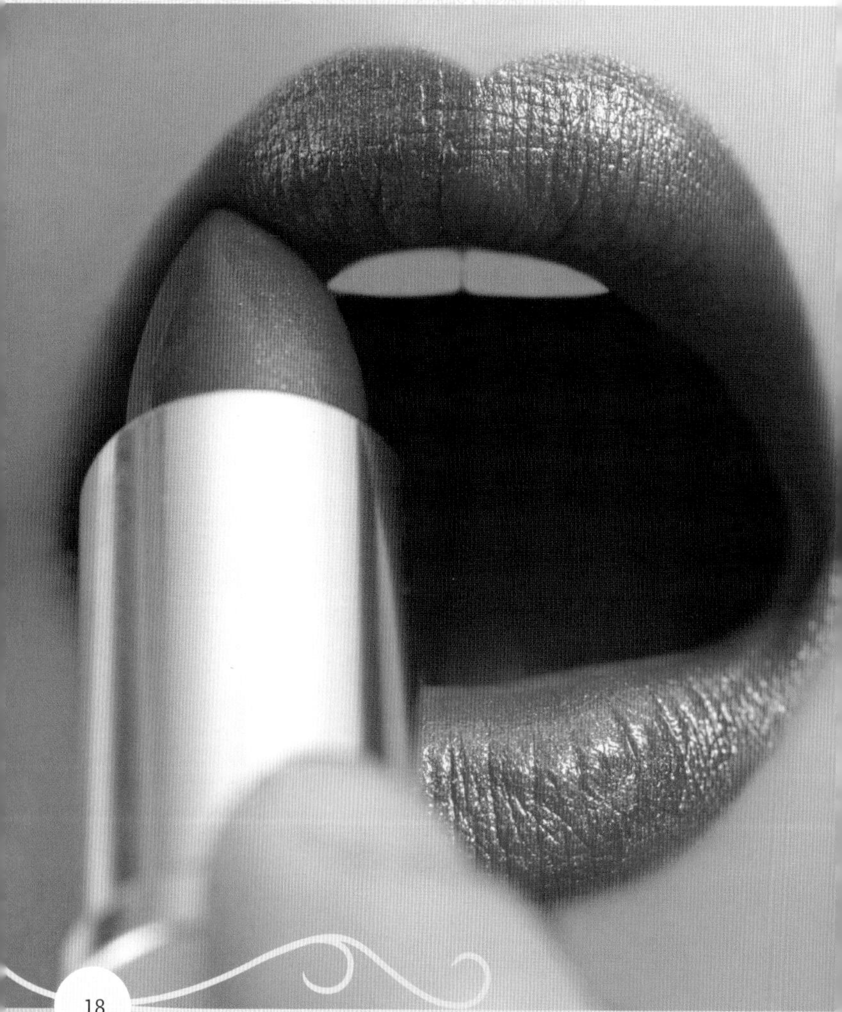

4. Luscious lips

Want plump, bee-stung, kissable lips? Before facing the needle try a few simple tips on how to fake them.

We can't all do pillar-box lips. Bold colours emphasise less than perfect lips but if you haven't the colouring or the requisite attitude, red lipstick can look more hooker than siren. Still, there's plenty you can do to enhance your pout.

Size up your lips

Assess their shape. You can minimise a large mouth and lips that are too full by choosing a neutral tone of lipstick. Use a lipliner to draw a line just inside the lips and choose a dark shade of lipstick to fill, which will help to make them look smaller. Stay clear of dark colours if your lips are thin, as they'll make them look even smaller. Instead, use a lipliner to draw a line just over your natural lip line to create the illusion of fuller lips and then go for a bright colour to plump them up even more. Glossy or pearl lipsticks can also make lips look fuller, as they reflect the light.

Here's an idea for you...

To get whiter-looking teeth go for berries, plums and blue-based red lipsticks. The contrast will help make your teeth appear whiter and brighter. Avoid any yellow- or orange-based shades, including corals and browny colours, as they can make your teeth look yellow.

Defining idea...

'Beauty, to me, is about being comfortable in your own skin. That, or a kick-ass red lipstick.'
GWYNETH PALTROW

Select the right shade of lippy

Experts say that olive skins look their best next to berry shades. If your complexion and hair are fair, stick to reds with pinkish undertones. If you have pale skin and dark hair you'll find that strong, bright-red lipstick can look amazing. And if your skin is dark, then pick deep, rich reds.

Pay your lips due service

Take the time to care for your lips in the same way that you care for your skin. Gently buff them with a soft, baby's toothbrush to remove dry skin and boost the circulation, then regularly apply lip balm. This is also a great way to soften up dry, cracked lips.

Try the bee-stung look

There's an art to perfecting bee-stung lips, so even those of us with thin lips can pout with the best of them. Try this:

1. First, outline your lips using a lip pencil in the same shade as your lipstick or lighter (never darker, unless you're a lap dancer or would like to be mistaken for one).

2. Then, using a lip brush, 'fill in' your lips. Instead of using a block of matt colour, build up gradually using a sheer lipstick. That way you'll capture the light, which will make your lips look fuller and plumper. Using a highlighter pen, draw a fine line around your upper lip, just above your Cupid's bow. Alternatively, try blending little dots of reflective foundation on your upper lip, which will also help accentuate a natural pout.

3. Finish with a dab of lipgloss on the fullest part of your lips.

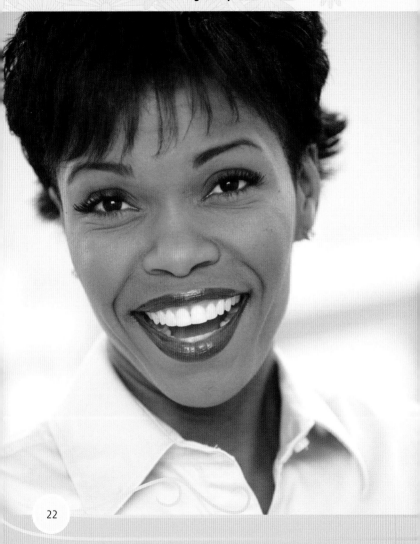

5. Great gnashers

Confidence, good looks and success are the kind of qualities a brilliant smile can impart. Dig out that floss today.

I've always been a bit obsessed with teeth, as I had braces as a child. A full Hannibal Lecter number that tortured my poor wayward teeth into meek submission and earned me odd stares on the school bus.

As a result, I notice every detail about someone's smile – veneers, caps, chips, crowns, the works. I assess the teeth of everyone I meet with my own kind of Playtex barometer: 'has she or hasn't she?' When British starlets go off to Hollywood in search of stardom and come back with newly bleached, chiselled, perfected teeth it's as obvious to me as if they'd come back with a third breast.

Being a teeth person, I look at people with a naturally beautiful smile with awe. It's the first thing I notice about someone. Imperfect teeth can make the seemingly beautiful less so. And a gorgeous set of pearlies can transform the merely plain into a radiant beauty. Psychologists say this is quite a normal reaction. Apparently, we assign negative character traits to people with a bad dental appearance.

Having a pleasant smile makes you appear not just more attractive, but also more honest and trustworthy. And when you smile a beautiful smile, you make the person you're smiling at feel better and generate warmth, happiness and confidence.

Here's an idea for you...

Stained teeth? Try this the old wives' tale: add a drop of clove oil to your toothpaste before brushing your teeth to help brighten your smile.

Your teeth can even make you look younger. Anthropologists say that this is because white and even teeth, healthy pink gums and a convex smile are characteristics of youth. However, as the years go by, our teeth lose their luminosity and become dull, stained and chipped. A mouthful of fillings can also make your smile look dull and grinding your teeth can wear them down. So, taking care of them and investing in the odd procedure (whitening, straightening, etc.) can actually take years off you.

Considering all these plus points, it's little wonder that we're spending a fortune on our teeth these days and that there's a cosmetic dentist on every high street. To keep your teeth looking their best try the following:

✿ Dentists say it's vital to use a meticulous cleaning routine and to use the best tooth products you can. Brush your teeth at least twice a day and ideally after each meal.
✿ Make sure you visit your dentist regularly – at least every 12 months – and never miss a check up.
✿ If needs be, invest in cosmetic procedures or braces. Amazing techniques are available these days and full-on braces are a thing of the past.
✿ Floss at least once a day.
✿ Cut down on sugary snacks and try fruit, vegetables and calcium-rich low-fat yoghurt instead. If you must eat something sweet stick to chocolate, as with chewy sweets the sugar gets sloshed around in your mouth for longer.

✿ Finish meals with cheese, which helps neutralise the acid in your mouth and therefore helps prevent tooth decay. Cheese is rich in calcium and phosphorous and this helps replace some of the minerals in tooth enamel, thereby strengthening teeth.

✿ Chew gum. Look for brands that contain xylitol because it's been found to help protect against – even reverse – tooth decay. Xylitol is found naturally in berries, mushrooms, lettuce and corn on the cob, too.

✿ Avoid stain-causing culprits such as coffee, tea, cigarettes and red wine. Try a whitening toothpaste to brighten your smile and have your teeth cleaned by a hygienist every six months.

Defining idea...

'A smile is an inexpensive way to change your looks.'
CHARLES GORDY, author

Are you brushing correctly? And for long enough? In order to clean all your tooth surfaces thoroughly you need to spend at least two minutes at it each time. The brushing motion itself helps remove stains, so don't cheat!

✿ First, focus on the inner and outer surfaces of your teeth. Place your toothbrush at a 45-degree angle and use gentle, short, tooth-wide strokes following your gum line. To clean the inside surfaces of front teeth, tilt your brush vertically and use gentle up-and-down strokes with the toe of your brush.

✿ Then move on to your chewing surfaces, holding your brush flat and brushing back and forth.

✿ Next, brush your tongue. Use a back-to-front sweeping method to remove food particles, which will also help freshen your mouth.

✿ Finally, gently brush the roof of the mouth.

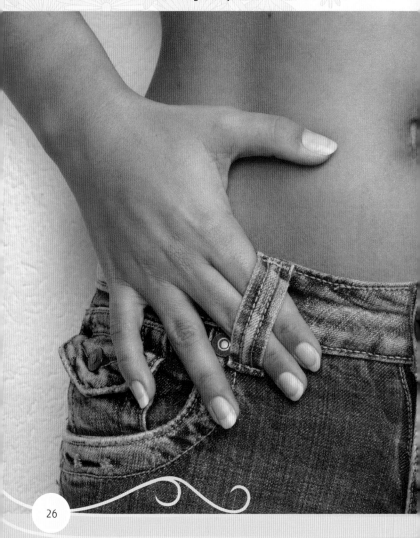

6. Beat the bloat

Bloating is the bane of many women's lives. It can add pounds overnight, immediately limit your fashion choices and force you to resort to your 'fat' wardrobe. Fortunately, you can beat it.

You know how it is. When your stomach is firm and flat the world seems a kinder, brighter place. You can slip effortlessly into jeans, flattering black dresses do actually flatter you and bikinis become less frightening.

Bloating is caused by trapped wind in your digestive system. The chief culprits range from food intolerances, constipation, too much alcohol, too much salt, eating too quickly or munching on too many gas-causing foods such as baked beans. Many women suffer premenstrual bloating too. And even stress can be to blame. Here are some ways to deflate that protruding tummy:

- ✿ Cut down on top bloaters such as wheat and replace them with rice or oats, which are usually better tolerated. Swap bran cereals for corn cereals, or breakfast on fresh fruit and yoghurt instead.
- ✿ Avoid constipation by eating plenty of fresh fruit and vegetables and drinking plenty of fluids. Also, go to the loo when you get the urge; resisting can muck up your digestive system further.
- ✿ Try a course of probiotics (acidophilus), which can help rebalance the good and bad bacteria in your digestive system. If the balance gets

Here's an idea for you...

Stress can play havoc with your digestive system so aim to set aside plenty of time for quality rest and relaxation and develop some great strategies for nipping stress in the bud.

out of kilter your system will slow down, which can cause lots of gas in your gut. You can buy supplements from the chemist or eat a bio yoghurt or yoghurt-based drink everyday.

✿ Fill your fruit bowl. Apples, pears and rhubarb are a great source of potassium, which helps rebalance your body's fluid levels. They're also a good source of pectin, a soluble fibre that keeps you regular. Other good non-bloaters are cherries and citrus fruit. Pineapples are great for beating bloat, too, as they contain the wonder-enzyme bromelain that helps digestion, alleviates wind and can soothe your stomach. Fresh pineapple is better than tinned, which tends to lose much of its bromelain. Try papaya, too, which contains enzymes such as papain that can be good for your digestion, particularly if you've been eating lots of rich meaty foods.

✿ Cut down on alcohol and salty foods, which can cause fluid retention and inflate that bloated tummy further. That's because your body holds on to fluid to dilute the extra salt. Avoid adding salt to your meals, but also cut back on ready meals and processed foods, which often contain tons of salt. Try cooking from scratch more often so you can keep your eye on your salt intake.

✿ Eat plenty of natural diuretics to help beat water retention, including celery, onion, parsley, coffee, tea, aubergine (eggplant), garlic and peppermint.

✿ Check you're eating enough protein like fish, lean meat or tofu, as nutrition experts say protein can also reduce fluid retention. But, don't overdo the beans or pulses as they can make matters worse.

✿ Address those PMS symptoms and if you're plagued with bloating each month, try a supplement. There's evidence that taking 1,000 mg of calcium a day (the recommended daily allowance is 700 mg) may improve problems concerning water retention. Try evening primrose oil and vitamin B6 supplements too to help minimise those grim PMS symptoms.

✿ Drink at least eight glasses of water a day. Regular, small amounts are best.

✿ Slow down at mealtimes, stop eating on the run and aim to savour your food and chew everything thoroughly. When you gulp your meals down you can swallow air, which can bloat you.

✿ Try some tummy-toning moves. Pilates is a great way to work your stomach muscles. It gave me abs of steel in just a few weeks when I first discovered it. It really helps pull your stomach up and in and is a great way to get your waist back after having a baby.

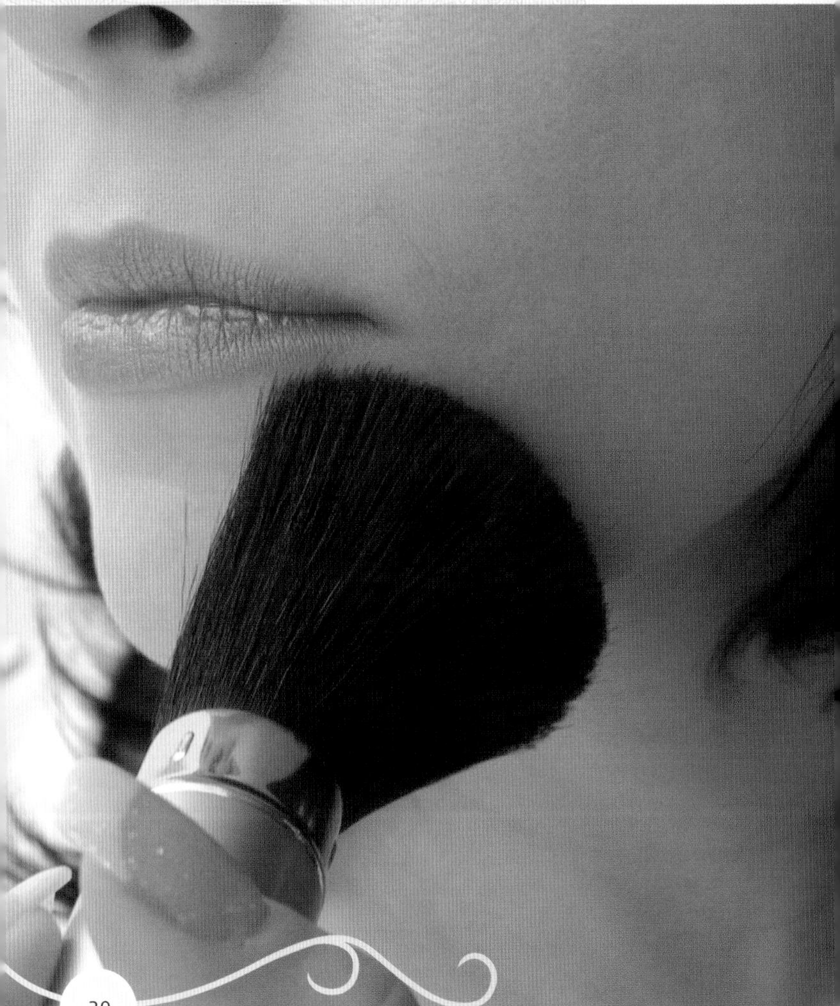

7. Fabulous foundations

Beautiful skin can be a sign of youth, good health, meticulous grooming, great genes or a combination of these. If you fall short in any department, you'll want to know how to get it out of a bottle.

A beauty counter is like an Aladdin's cave or a knicker draw: full of pretty things, yet you're really only interested in finding an item that works miracles.

Everyone knows that good skin stems from drinking lots of water, getting plenty of sleep and eating a healthy diet high in fruit and vegetables. If you're short on time, however, and haven't been all that saintly, you'll want results and you'll want them now. The key, as we all know, is to look natural, but not too natural.

Fortunately, these days foundations contain all sorts of silicone powders and light-diffusing pigments to disguise flaws and make skin glow. They've also been imbued with great sunscreens and vitamins to protect skin from the sun. And there are mattifying formulations to help even out skin tone.

How to apply the no make-up look

Gone are the days of Barbara Cartland-style make-up – trowelled on and proud of it. In fact, these days experts advise using foundation only where you need it, i.e. the often oily T-zone (forehead, nose and chin)

31

Here's an idea for you...

If you've got open pores or spots, in the daytime avoid using bronzers containing shimmery particles that will draw attention to them. Save these bronzers for evenings, when the light will be on your side and you'll look sexy and sultry. For daytime pick matt bronzing powders.

and under the eyes. You may not need to apply foundation everywhere, but make sure you blend carefully, nay obsessively, into the skin, especially around nostrils, the sides of the nose and corners of the eyes. Beauticians recommend oil-free or matt formulas for oily skin, rich moisturising foundations for dry skin and stick or compacts for combination skin.

If you're trying to disguise broken veins on your skin, use a concealer that is one shade lighter than your skin tone, then dust with powder. Be sure to add concealer after foundation and not before else you'll wipe it away. If you have wrinkles or spots I suggest you steer away from heavy matt foundations, as sheer coverage is actually more flattering. And if you're prone to acne, avoid the compact foundations that are applied with a sponge, which attract bacteria that can make spots worse. Remember, you don't always need to splash out on concealer, just use the drier bit of foundation in the cap to cover blemishes.

Make-up by numbers

1. Start by moisturising your skin well, then leave it for a few minutes to let the moisture sink into your skin. If you're using an eye cream, now's the time to apply it. Foundation can often crease under eyes, which can be ageing.

2. Pour a penny-sized amount of
    foundation into your palm then
    dot it over your forehead, nose,
    cheeks and chin. Using your
    fingers or a sponge, blend it
    gently outwards using small strokes. Don't forget to sweep foundation
    over eyelids too; it can make a great base for eyeshadow. You're aiming
    to make the foundation disappear into the hairline and jawline. If you've
    been too heavy handed, dab the surplus away with a clean damp
    sponge. Always put your foundation on in good light and think blend,
    blend, blend.

    Defining idea...

    **'The best thing is to look natural, but it
    takes make-up to look natural.'**
    CALVIN KLEIN

3. Next focus on concealing blemishes such as spots and under-eye lines.
    Dot concealer over the areas you want to cover using a fingertip or tiny
    brush and blend well.

4. Now 'set' the foundation by dusting powder lightly over your T-zone
    (if you're using a light-diffusing foundation you won't need this as
    you're aiming for a dewy rather than matt look). Blot your face after
    applying powder so it doesn't lie on your face – never put powder
    under your eyes as it can accentuate fine lines. Always avoid thick
    bases as they're ageing too.

5. Then add blusher onto the apples of the cheeks. To find the apples
    suck your cheeks in and smile.

6. If you're going for the nude look, make sure you add plenty of
    mascara otherwise your eyes may 'disappear'. Use brown or black
    mascara and eyeliner to define your eyes.

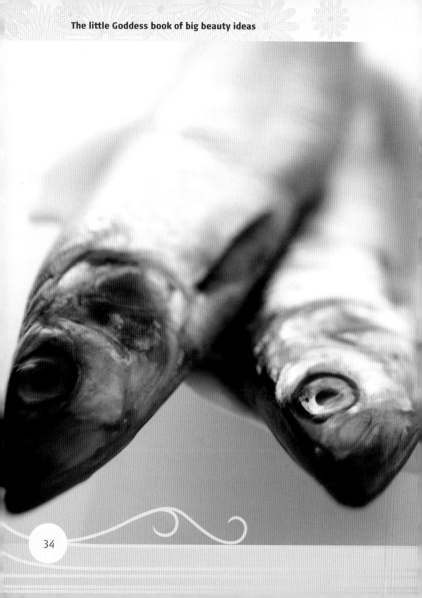

8. Feed your face

When it comes to your complexion, diet can be far more valuable than make-up. Here's your guide to what to eat today for glowing, less troublesome skin tomorrow.

Experts tell us that diet can help fight certain skin conditions. For instance, oily fish alleviates the symptoms of psoriasis, and scientists have found a link between refined carbohydrates and acne. Brightly coloured fruit and vegetables can also reduce sun damage.

You know yourself that eating nothing but junk will take its toll on your face. Think about your most recent wild evening on the town. Perhaps it involved a couple of cocktails and a bottle of wine, followed by something greasy, salty and bursting with additives? How did your skin look the morning after? Pasty, dull and grey? The good news is that you can dramatically change your complexion in days simply by cutting out the rubbish and filling up on some skin-friendly foods.

So, what to eat? Well, omega-3 fatty acids, found in fish, for example, have good anti-inflammatory action and are great for improving the elasticity and texture of skin. And fruit and vegetables are rich in antioxidants that help fight the free radicals caused by pollution, sun and cigarette smoke that can lead to wrinkles. Free radicals not only cause cancer and heart disease, they can also wreak havoc on skin by

Here's an idea for you...

Patchouli is an essential oil thought to be good for skin as it can encourage the production of new skin cells. Add a few drops to your bath or mix three drops with 10 ml of a carrier oil such as sweet almond and give yourself a gentle massage.

damaging your cell membranes and the connective tissues that support it. Certain foods can help boost circulation too, including onions, garlic, nuts, pumpkin seeds and fish. When your blood is circulating at optimum levels, it means that your cells – including your skin cells – are getting a regular supply of life-giving nutrients and oxygen.

Get a skinful

- ✿ **Fish** Oily fish such as sardines, mackerel and salmon are rich in fatty acids.
- ✿ **Turkey** A great source of lean protein, essential for making collagen. It also contains an amino acid known as carnosine, which can help prevent wrinkles.
- ✿ **Nuts** Packed with omega-3 fatty acids, which help control the lipids and fats in your body that can help skin stay soft and smooth. They're also rich in skin-friendly vitamin E. Brazil nuts contain the antioxidant selenium, which helps fight free radicals.
- ✿ **Spinach** Particularly rich in vitamin K, which is good for blood circulation, making sure nutrients and oxygen reach every cell. It's also rich in antioxidants.

- ✿ **Berries** Bursting with antioxidants.
- ✿ **Citrus fruit** Rich in vitamin C, which can help maintain the structure of collagen and help repair cuts and grazes.
- ✿ **Avocados** Rich in vitamin E and healthy monounsaturated fats.
- ✿ **Sweet potatoes** Rich in vitamins C and E, which help fight free radicals and may help prevent sun damage.
- ✿ **Pumpkin seeds** Packed with omega-3 fatty acids. They're also a good source of vitamin E, which is good for skin firmness.
- ✿ **Cruciferous vegetables** Broccoli, cauliflower, cabbage, etc., are rich in antioxidants and fibre, good for keeping your digestive system working properly and for stimulating the liver, which helps removes waste and toxins from the body. When you reduce your toxic load, your skin looks better.
- ✿ **Kiwi fruit** Rich in vitamin C, which helps build collagen and strengthens capillaries. They're also full of beta-carotene, which helps fight cell-damaging free radicals.
- ✿ **Water** At least eight glasses a day. Helps metabolise fat, reduces puffiness and helps your body flush waste from its cells.

The bad guys

- ✿ **Cakes, biscuits, white bread, etc.** Studies show a link between high intakes of refined starchy carbohydrates and acne. These foods also make your skin puffy, dehydrated and prone to allergic reactions.

Defining idea...

**'Our food choices have everything to do
with how we look and affect wrinkles, skin
tone, eye bags and puffiness, and facial
vibrancy and clarity.'**

DR NICHOLAS PERRICONE, dermatologist
and author

✿ **Sugary foods** Can raise your blood sugar, which interferes with the way the hormone insulin behaves, making it flood your body with excess glucose. This causes collagen fibres to bunch up and results in loss of firmness and deep wrinkles.

✿ **Salty foods** Salt can cause fluid retention, which can make you look puffy and bloated and cause eye bags.

✿ **Coffee** Can dehydrate your body, leading to dark circles and puffiness.

✿ **Alcohol** Can increase the number of free radicals in your body and dehydrate your skin.

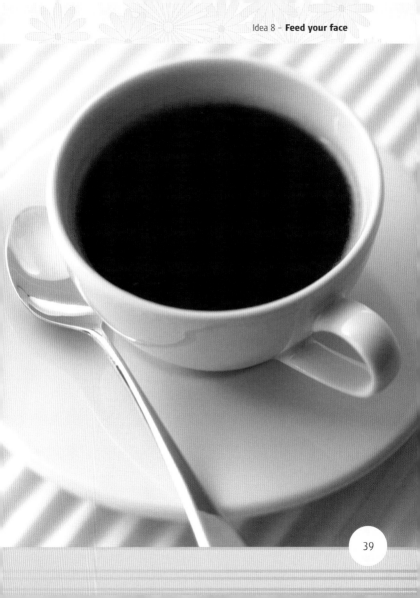

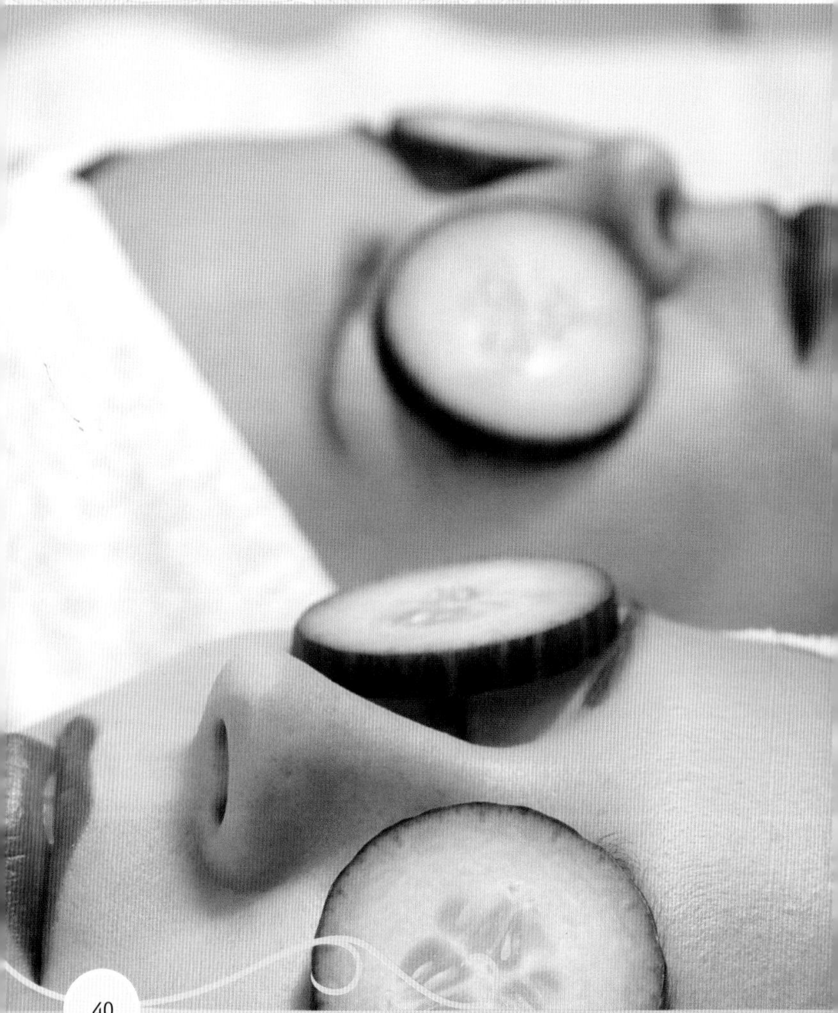

9. Quick fixes

Puffy eyes? Dark circles? Frizzy hair? Try these instant beautifiers for those hot date emergencies.

You know how it is. A huge bouquet of plump pink roses lands on your desk at work with a note saying, 'Darling, meet me at Claridges at eight. Wear something irresistible.'

In my dreams! Nevertheless, there *are* moments when we need to look super-gorgeous fast, like for a last-minute party, date or business lunch, for example. And since they'll undoubtedly arise on a bad nail, spot or hair day, here are some troubleshooting tips to catch the beauty demons off guard.

Cover up those spots

First, clean the spot area using cotton wool and a medicated lotion. Next, apply a mattifying product or gel to the area to remove any excess oil and prevent your concealer from sliding off. Pick a concealer that's the same colour as your face, ideally dry in texture rather than creamy, and apply it right in the middle of the spot. Using a brush or your middle finger, wipe away any excess. Remember, you're trying to camouflage the spot, not the area around it.

Here's an idea for you...

For posh nails cut corners with press-on falsies. Pick the pre-glued ones and simply press them on over your natural nails. They should last up to three days.

Instantly boost your complexion

Exfoliating to remove the layer of dead skin cells that dulls your complexion is the easiest way to brighten your skin and make you feel perkier. Splashing your face with cold water is a great pick-me-up, too. Beauty doyenne Eve Lom (www.evelom.co.uk) has her own method. Start by massaging in a rich oil-based cleanser and then remove it using a muslin cloth. Next, massage cleanser over your face and neck gently, applying deep pressure with the pads of your fingertips. Start behind the ears to stimulate the lymphatic system, relieve congestion and reduce fluid. Repeat this three times, then rinse the cloth, rub off the cleanser and splash your face with cold water.

Fix puffy eyes

Give yourself a mini lymphatic drainage massage to help beat the fluid retention. Tap your middle finger around each eye in circular movements, then lie down and place cotton wool pads soaked in witch hazel or rosewater over your eyes. Alternatively, try damp camomile teabags that have been cooled in the fridge. Drink plenty of water too as dehydration can make puffy eyes worse. If you've time a quick workout can help boost circulation and lymph drainage. As a long-term solution, sleep with your head raised higher than your body.

Brighten dark circles

These nasties occur when your
blood vessels become visible
through your skin. Some people
have naturally thin skin, but you do lose fat in this area as you age, so
they tend to get worse. Start in the corner of your eye and apply
concealer a shade lighter than your skin tone. Ideally, choose cream
concealer as it's easier to apply and goes on more evenly. Some experts
say that eye creams containing vitamin K, which helps boost blood flow,
can help with dark circles.

Tame frizziness

You may have been born with frizzy hair. Or too much sun, too many
colourants, blow-drying at too high a temperature and the need for a
jolly good trim have left it crispy or wayward. Aim to condition your hair
regularly and book that haircut if it's overdue. If you're on the point of
going out use a leave-in conditioner before you blow-dry or add a few
drops of smoothing serum that contains panthenol or silicone-based
products to coat the cuticle and help it lie flat. Don't be afraid to spritz
your hair with hairspray either as it will help prevent moisture in humid
air (which causes your hair to frizz) from penetrating your hair.

Defining idea...

'Illusions are the mirages of Hope.'
ANONYMOUS

Defining idea...

Glam up your hair

Try this super speedy blow-dry. Lightly spray your hair with water then add a root-lifting product to give you instant body and volume. Start by blow-drying your roots, lifting the hair upwards as you go. Then smooth your hair into style using a natural bristle brush to give you extra shine. Finally, use your fingers to tousle your hair into a dishevelled but glam style, spray some perfume in the air and 'walk' into it. Instant gorgeousness.

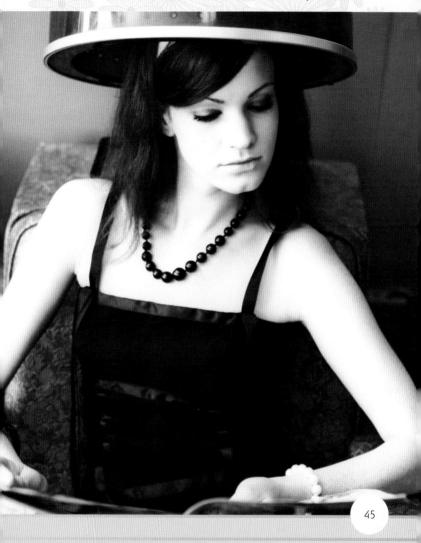

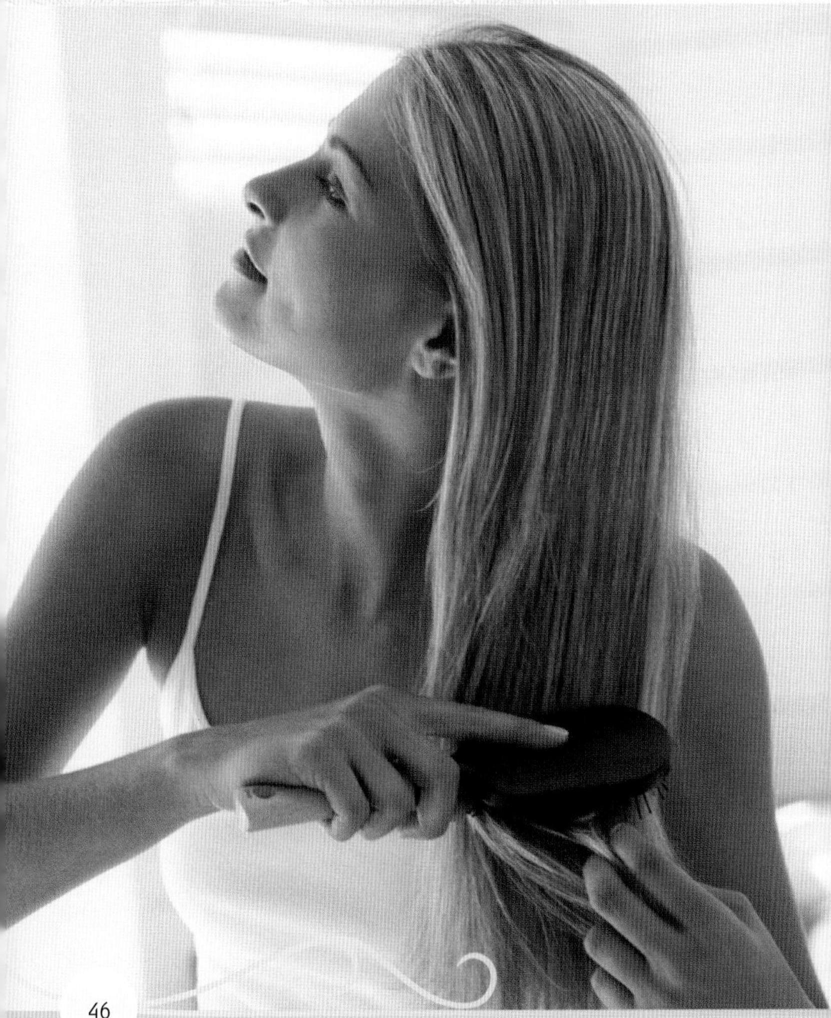

10. Clever hair care

Simple tricks to turn a bad hair day good, plus hairdos to knock years off you.

Genetics, weather, hormones, diet and hair products (too many, not enough or the wrong type) can all take their toll. If you're frizzy, flat or frumpy, you need some professional help.

We've done the legwork for you, so try these invaluable solutions to everyday hair headaches.

Book that trim

A regular trim – every six to eight weeks – really is the best way to keep your hair in tip-top condition. Each hair on your head grows at its own pace, so within weeks they can look uneven and scraggly. Split ends happen when the individual layers of hair shafts separate due to chemicals, weather or too much heat from styling. You can help to seal split ends by using a leave-in conditioner, but the effect will only be temporary. Your hair grows between a third and half an inch per month, so you'll recover the length again in no time. A trim will make your hair look thicker, healthier and glossier.

Defining idea...

'I'm not offended by all the dumb-blonde jokes because I know that I'm not dumb. I also know I'm not blonde.'
DOLLY PARTON

Here's an idea for you...

Put your hair in a high ponytail and you'll look years younger. It will help lift your face. A fringe can knock years off you too, plus it can emphasise your cheekbones. And highlights around your face are anti-ageing as they lighten and brighten your complexion.

The best blow-dry

✿ Blot wet hair first with a towel. If your hair is fine, only condition the ends because if you put it on the roots you'll make it lank. Spray some gel onto the roots and spread it evenly by rubbing with your fingers. To control frizz, use a small dollop of smoothing balm rather than gel, which can make hair drier.

✿ For added volume, use a handful of mousse about the size of a golf ball. Also, try wrapping the top layers of your hair around two large Velcro rollers when your hair is 95% dry and then finish blow-drying.

✿ Wait until your hair is quite dry before you blow-dry it and you'll do less damage; hair can lose up to 30% of its moisture when blow-dried.

✿ Clip your hair up into sections. Start with the hair at the back of your head first, then the side sections. Pull each section taut with a large round brush and dry from the root to the tip. Use the nozzle to tuck the ends under or to lift hair from the roots for volume.

✿ After drying each section, give it a blast of cold air to help 'set' the hair.

✿ When you hair is totally dry, part it. Now's the time to add a bit of serum to coarse, long or curly hair. Otherwise, wait until the hair is cool then spritz your hands with hairspray and rub it over your hair.

Tips for curly or frizzy hair

Frizz is the result of too much heat, sun or chemicals used to bleach, colour, straighten or curl your hair.

Defining idea...

'Hair style is the final tip-off whether or not a woman really knows herself.'
HUBERT DE GIVENCHY

❀ Choose conditioners with panthenol and silicone, which make the cuticle lie flat and make hair look smoother and sleeker.

❀ If you have naturally wiry or wispy hair, always use conditioner after shampooing and also invest in a deep-conditioning product. Also, wash your hair thoroughly to get rid of traces of shampoo and conditioner; otherwise it'll look lank. You'll know when you've washed away the last of the residue because when you run your hand through your hair, it should feel squeaky-clean.

❀ Never use too much conditioner even if your hair is thick. The right size for shoulder length hair is that of an almond, less if it's shorter.

❀ Blot hair with a towel to absorb excess moisture. A wide-toothed comb can detangle curly hair without tearing it and help to eliminate frizz. Anything else can break or tear your hair, leaving it with split ends.

❀ Apply a protective product before you blow-dry to prevent hair from dehydrating and then use a diffuser and your fingers to gently blow-dry. Avoid brushes or combs, as they'll just make your hair frizz. After drying, rub a few drops of serum into the palms of your hands then smooth it over your hair to calm wayward strands and seal in moisture.

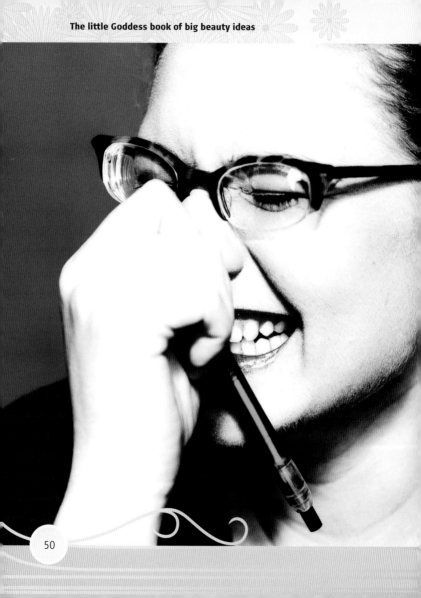

11. The power of vitality

Discover the secret of that special joie de vivre that will make your eyes sparkle and your entire body radiate gorgeousness.

You can be dolled up to the nines, having just stepped out of the salon, but if you're feeling lacklustre you're simply not going to look your best.

One dictionary definition of vitality is 'the power of remaining alive, vigorous; liveliness, energy, durability'. Personally I think it's a combination of energy, liveliness and a passion for living that comes with seeing the best in everything and seeking out life's greatest sensations. It's about sensual pleasures – things that look, sound, taste, smell and feel great yet aren't too calorie-laden or illegal.

Here are a few vitality secrets to try today.

Initiate sex more
One study showed that people who had sex three times a week looked considerably younger than people who had it less often. Sex is great for your circulation, can release feel-good endorphins to keep you feeling happy and can help strengthen your bond with your partner.

Eat delicious foods
Choose healthy and decadent goodies such as artichokes, plump strawberries, huge asparagus tips and the finest organic chocolate.

Here's an idea for you...

Make your own pick-me-up CD or tape. Pick your favourite energising and uplifting pieces of music and play them in the car, as you walk in the park or before that scary meeting. Instant joy!

Research shows that men prefer normal-sized women with big, hearty appetites so combine this with the previous tip.

Exercise regularly

Dance, run or swim three times a week – anything that involves moving your body is great for you. After twenty minutes of exercise, your body produces endorphins. Exercise is also great for your self-confidence and body image.

Go out to play

Indulge in regular girly rituals; take long soaks in delicious-smelling candlelit baths, splurge on a pedicure, wear flimsy strappy summer dresses, teeter around in an expensive pair of heels or have a pampering party night in with your friends.

Get out more

Get outdoors – it's a surefire mood booster. Surround yourself with greenery; make a window box and fill your home with flowers. Studies show fresh cut flowers in the office can boost productivity, too.

Perk up your extremities

Sore, aching feet squeezed into impractical shoes can radiate up your legs and make you generally sore and miserable. Treat yourself to a reflexology treatment or a darn good pedicure. Or try an Indian head massage; it's

relaxing, energising and you can
do it in your lunch hour.

Surround yourself with beautiful things

Splurge on a beautiful picture,
spend a day at a gallery or museum
or buy tickets to the opera or
ballet. Think of it as a spiritual facial.

Cut down on chemicals

Chemicals can put your body under stress and rob you of energy. Hoover
regularly, use a water filter, hang your washing to dry outside, eat
organic when you can afford it and use chemical-free household
products where you can.

Clean up your house

Decluttering has an amazingly positive impact on energy levels. Start
small and devote just twenty minutes a day on a shelf, drawer or
cupboard. And be brutal; if you haven't worn or used something for six
months, get rid of it.

Inhale mind-sharpening scents

Pine, peppermint, eucalyptus and
jasmine are known to stimulate
the part of your brain that makes
you alert.

Defining idea...

*'There is a vitality, a life force, an energy, a
quickening, that is translated through you
into action, and because there is only one
of you in all time, this expression is
unique.'*
MARTHA GRAHAM

Defining idea...

'Energy is eternal delight.'
WILLIAM BLAKE

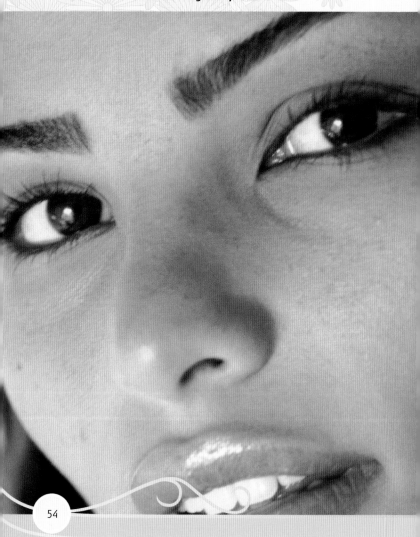

12. Enhance your eyes

They're said to be the windows to the soul, the first thing people notice and capable of disarming a man at 100 paces. But what if your eyes are more Mole Man than Bette Davis?

According to anthropologists, the most attractive women's faces are 'child-like', with smooth skin, a peaches-and-cream complexion, a small nose and big eyes with long Bambi lashes.

These are all good reasons to take care of your eyes. Easy-peasy eye care includes taking off your eye make-up every night, keeping dirty hankies or fingers away from them and patting instead of rubbing the skin surrounding them. Make sure you get lots of sleep, drink gallons of water, apply a regular dab of eye cream and treat yourself to the odd cucumber or teabag session.

As for making them bigger and veiled in long, thick, fluttery eyelashes, you'll need a few good tools and clever make-up techniques.

Try these:

✿ Start with your eyebrows and pluck any stray hairs with a pair of tweezers.

Here's an idea for you...

Bring out the colour of your eyes using contrasts. Pinks, mauves and greys look great on blue eyes. Or use really dark colours for stunning contrasts. Avoid pinks if your eyes are red and tired; stick to neutrals or ivories instead. Remember: blend, blend, blend.

❀ Apply a pale or neutral colour over the upper eyelid, blending over the outer edges, to give a good matt base on which you can blend and build darker and stronger colours. Even a dab of foundation can create a great base for colour and cover any redness or blotchiness.

❀ Apply a brown or grey eyeshadow, from the middle to the outer edge of the eye. Start with a tiny bit of colour and add more layers, blending as you go.

❀ Brush a thin line of a darker shade along the upper lid. Add a little shading under the eye, too, at the outer edge.

❀ Using white pencil along the lower inner socket of your eyes can make them more striking. Or dot a tiny spot of white shadow in the inner corners of your eyes to make them look wider apart.

❀ If your eyes are small, remember that you'll make them look even smaller by using eyeshadow or eyeliner around the entire eye as this will effectively close them up.

❀ False eyelashes can really open up the eyes so don't be afraid of them. Try a few individual lashes on the outer corner of the eye, then add a few shorter ones, and alternate between the two as you work towards the middle of the eye.

❀ Invest in eyelash curlers, which really help to open your eyes. They're easier to use than they look, too. Just hold them so that your upper lashes lie between the two rims, then squeeze and roll upwards.

Defining idea...

'Cosmetics is a boon to every woman, but a girl's best beauty aid is still a near-sighted man.'
YOKO ONO

❀ Eyeshadow spillage? Before you start, pop a layer of translucent loose powder underneath each eye to catch any of the eyeshadow that falls on your cheeks. You can then simply brush it away and you don't have to reapply foundation.

❀ Stick to black mascara for drama, brown if you're very blonde, or try the 'no make-up' look, which is also more flattering against older skins.

❀ Some make-up artists recommend you put mascara on the top lashes only and leave the bottom ones bare – it makes you look brighter and less tired.

❀ Don't dismiss coloured mascara. Try navy blue (not electric blue) to make the whites of your eyes look whiter, or plum, which can look great on blondes.

❀ Avoid putting powder underneath your eyes, as when it 'cakes' it shows up every crease and fine line and can be very ageing.

❀ How many layers of mascara? Ideally two for maximum drama, but don't let it dry between layers or it may cake and flake.

❀ Invest in eyedrops, a great way to put a sparkle in your eye.

13. Photogenic fakes: looking great in photos

You know who they are – the plain Janes and Johns who somehow look like film stars when they're captured on camera. You can join them.

Models and celebrities know all the tricks of the trade – if you watch them carefully at red carpet events you'll catch them strike a carefully calculated pose as the paparazzi gather. So, next time you have to face your public, try some of these tricks picked up from celebrities and photographers.

✿ To look your slimmest try standing with one foot slightly in front of the other, and gently pivot on your feet so that your body including your shoulders are at a slight angle. Putting your hands on your hips can make your waist look smaller, so overall it'll take inches off your body.

✿ If you're sitting down, just lean forward and rest your elbows on your knees – you'll disguise any wobbly thighs and look slimmer.

✿ Look lively. Greta Garbo *froideur* isn't always the most flattering attitude to adopt in snaps. In fact, some professional portrait photographers insist the best pictures are always taken when the subject is looking animated and chipper – that way the subject's personality is captured. You can still engineer your 'best side' in front of the camera.

✿ Practise in the mirror. If you find a pose you're happy with, it's worth perfecting it, so you can strike it the moment the camera comes out.

✿ Brighten up. Dark colours can be slimming, but black can be draining against the face, so choose brighter colours on your top half to enhance your skin tone.

✿ Beware brightly patterned clothes; they can swamp you and detract from your face.

✿ Dark circles or bags under your eyes? Try lifting your chin – you'll avoid shadows falling on your face.

✿ Do smile. Forget looking moody – everyone actually looks more attractive when they're looking happy. Plus a lovely smile really does take the focus away from the bits you're less happy with.

✿ Poker straight hair can pull your face down. Putting your hair up can soften your features and draw attention to your smile.

Here's an idea for you...

Maximise your lips. To pout beautifully, try turning to the camera and saying 'Wogan'. Sounds bizarre, granted, but try it. It somehow produces the perfect pout – glamour models swear by it.

✿ Get them to take more than one! The more photos you have taken, the more likely it is you'll be captured from a flattering angle. Remember, safety in numbers.

Make-up tricks

You'd be forgiven for thinking that slapping gallons of foundation and concealer over spots and blemishes would create alabaster skin and produce wonderful photographs you'd display with pride. Forget it: overdo the slap and you'll look like a waxwork – or, worse, a cross-dresser. Instead, be subtle.

Defining idea...

'With charm you've got to get up close to see it; style slaps you in the face.'
JOHN COOPER CLARKE, poet and comedian.

✿ Apply a light foundation only where necessary – sides of nose, over spots, that kind of thing.

✿ To avoid shiny-face, stick to matte formula make-up on your blemishes and only use creamy, reflective concealers on the eye.

✿ Flatter your best features – apply blush over to the apple part of your cheeks, sneak a couple of extra false lashes on your eyelids, slick on some glossy lipstick. Don't forget the golden rule of make-up, though: never overplay the eyes *and* the lips – choose between them before you open that make-up bag.

✿ Ask for a minute or two before the camera clicks so you can touch up and dab a bit of powder over shiny bits. Who cares if you seem vain – there are few things as insidious as unflattering photos of yourself *in someone else's hands...*

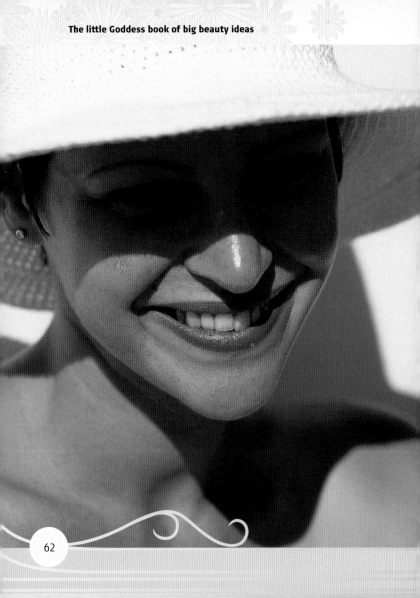

14. Save your skin

**A little bit of sun exposure can help you live longer –
but too much could kill you.**

It may seem unfair, but there isn't a more effective way of speeding up
the ageing process than lying on a sunlounger.

A glowing tan can cover a multitude of sins. Not only does the sun lead
to wrinkles which make us look older, it also damages the chromosomes
in our skin cells and can trigger skin cancer.

Ultraviolet light is the part of sunlight that damages skin. As UVB is 85%
responsible for burning the skin – and has traditionally been thought to
be the main cause of skin cancer – the first sunscreens mainly protected
against these rays. However, around fifteen years ago scientists began to
discover that UVA can also damage the skin in the longer term, by
causing the release of harmful free radicals in the skin. These can
suppress the immune system, cause allergic reactions such as prickly
heat and damage the DNA of skin cells. The result is premature ageing –
wrinkles, enlarged pores, bumps, pigmentation and saggy skin. There's
also growing evidence that it is mainly UVA rays that cause melanoma –
the most dangerous kind of skin cancer – and not UVB rays as was
originally thought.

Here's an idea for you...

Never know how much sunscreen is enough? A blob the size of a large coin should cover one arm and hand or your face and neck, and two blobs will do a leg and foot, your front torso or back. Sunscreen should be applied fifteen minutes before exposure, then reapplied immediately on exposure to the sun. Reapply every two hours as it gets rubbed off. And always reapply after swimming – even if it's a water-resistant sunscreen (they're designed to protect you while in the water but no sunscreen is completely waterproof, so a certain amount will come off). Try to wait five minutes after applying lotion before lying down – a protective film forms after five minutes so it's not as easily rubbed off. You'll need one 400 ml bottle of sunscreen per person for every ten days of a beach-based holiday.

But that doesn't mean avoiding the sun altogether – the body needs to be exposed to sunlight before it can make vitamin D, essential for strengthening the immune response, healthy bones and cardiovascular health. There's also been some interesting research recently into how sunlight affects our moods, and that exposure to natural light can stave off depression. This isn't a licence to strip off and bake yourself next summer. Just ten minutes outdoors every day, without sunblock, is enough sun exposure to allow your body to make vitamin D.

Nowadays, we're clued up about the dangers of sun exposure and most of us are aware of the basic rules to protect ourselves. But what is more worrying is that the risk of sun-related cancer is determined by how much exposure you received as a child; just one incidence of sunburn as a child more than doubles your odds of getting skin cancer and DNA damage to skin can result in cancer ten to thirty years on. It's

probably not what you want to
hear if you're part of the
generation who grew up accepting
that sunburn was a part of summer.
So what (if anything) can you do to
undo the damage of the past and
reduce your risk of skin cancer in
the future?

Defining idea...

**'Nobody grows old merely by living a
number of years. We grow old by deserting
our ideals. Years may wrinkle the skin, but
to give up enthusiasm wrinkles the soul.'**
Samuel Ullman, poet

You could start by drinking lots of green tea (around four cups a day).
Studies have also shown that compounds in green tea can fight skin
cancer. Stick with it – it's an acquired taste. Eating vegetables high in
beta-carotene and vitamin A such as carrots is also thought to protect
against skin cancers developing.

It's important to also keep an eye on your skin (and your partner's) –
75% of melanomas are spotted by individuals, not doctors, and with
early detection almost 100% of skin cancers are curable. See your doctor
immediately if an existing mole or dark patch is getting larger or a new
one is growing, if a mole has a ragged outline (ordinary moles are
smooth and regular) or if a mole has a mixture of different shades of
brown or black (ordinary moles may be dark brown but are all one
shade). You should also report the following changes if they don't
disappear within two weeks: an inflamed mole or one with a reddish
edge, one that starts to bleed, ooze or crust, a mole that changes
sensation or one that is substantially bigger than all of your other moles.

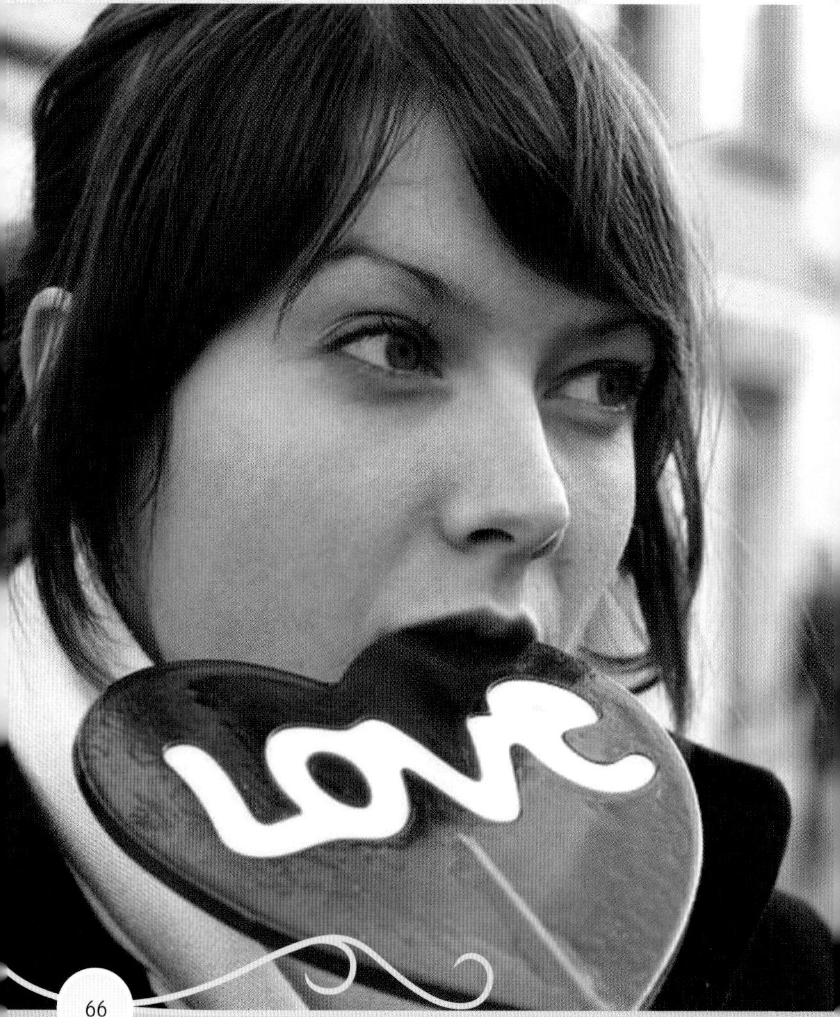
love

I want to be thin!

Are you an emotional eater?

When is food not food? When we start to get it mixed up with our best friend, looking to it for support and to make us feel better. Is your relationship with comfort food getting a bit too close for comfort? Respond to the following statements:

I eat when I'm not hungry:
Rarely/Sometimes/Often

If I have a bad morning ahead of me, I promise myself food as a reward:
Rarely/Sometimes/Often

Stressed out – and my first reaction is to turn to food:
Rarely/Sometimes/Often

I often think about my next meal when I've just eaten:
Rarely/Sometimes/Often

When I'm feeling low, foods 'call' to me and I can't think of anything else:
Rarely/Sometimes/Often

I'm always starting healthy eating habits or another diet, but even as I promise myself I'll change, I know I won't:
Rarely/Sometimes/Often

Which ideas do I need?

If you answered SOMETIMES 3 or more times, your attitude to food is ambivalent. Take the emotion out of food and see it for what it is – nourishing fuel. Understanding your energy needs will help, turn to idea 18, *Top gear*.

If you answered OFTEN 3 or more times, your attitude to food is as your best mate who will cheer you up when you're down. Food can't lift your mood in the long term. Turn to idea 22, *Are you an emotional eater?*, for more on curbing your cravings.

If you answered RARELY most of the time, your attitude is fine. If you're struggling on a diet, you might want to see idea 21, *It's never too late to change your mind*, on sticking to diets.

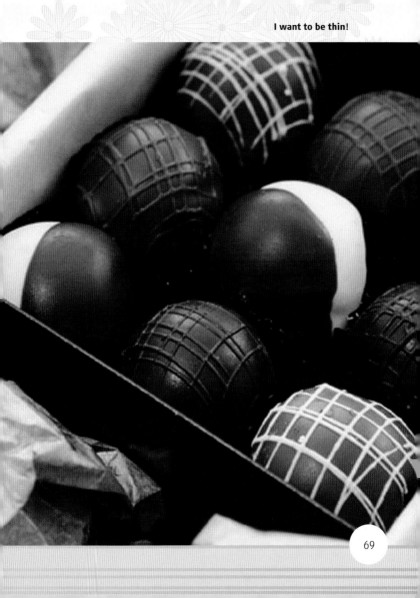

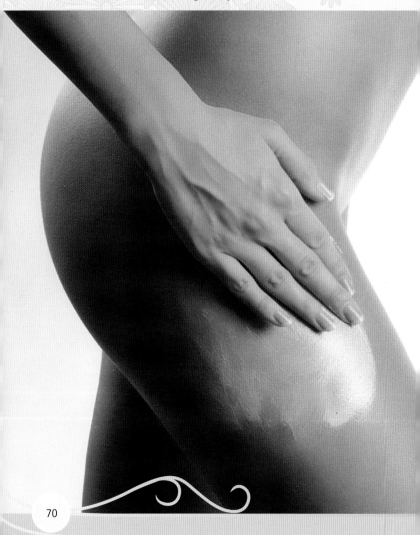

15. Bottom's up

Celebrate your curves. Having cellulite – as nearly nine out of ten women do – doesn't mean you can't feel gorgeous. Try some bottom pampering today.

The word cellulite was first coined back in the 70s, but it's no modern affliction. Just think of those Rubenesque lovelies, writhing about in the altogether. They'd never make the cover of today's Vogue, yet in their era they were considered the epitome of voluptuous sexiness.

Fashion has changed, and back in the days of yore, fatness (for that's essentially what cellulite is – body fat) would have been synonymous with wealth. Nowadays the smaller your thighs, the bigger your wallet. Women dread surplus pounds, aspiring instead to a neat peachy behind and racehorse legs. And cellulite, which becomes worse as you get older, is viewed as a sort of degenerative disease.

The truth is cellulite is just part of being a woman – 85–95% of us fall prey to it, including the world's most glamorous models and actresses.

There's nothing disease-like about it either: it's surplus fat held together by skin cells that have lost their elasticity. And it lurks about the areas of a woman's body that are designed to lay down fat – backs of thighs, bottoms, tummies, even your upper arms. The result? Fat cells squishing upwards against your skin and causing a cottage cheese effect – like stuffing bursting out of an old cushion.

Here's an idea for you...

Toning up your behind doesn't have to be a full-time occupation. Try this tiny bum-firming move which you can do anywhere. Raise one foot off the floor and kick it back behind you in tiny pulse-moves. Aim for 15 repetitions two or three times a day.

That's not to say you have to embrace cellulite as part of your femaleness (that's why we've written this book, after all). But before you get stressed, depressed and obsessed about the cellulitey bits, take a moment here to get a perspective, and to celebrate your curves.

A friend's husband once took a mould of her behind, which was, refreshingly, generously proportioned. He gave it to her as an anniversary present – a wonderful pumpkin of a bottom cast in bronze.

So the first lesson is 'remember, men love curves'. In fact men particularly love fleshy bottoms when they're paired with a small waist; studies show a waist/hip ratio of 0.7 is the magic formula most likely to get a man's pulse racing.

Don't forget too that your curves are there for a reason: making babies, having babies, feeding babies, filling out bikinis/ridiculously expensive undies, that sort of thing.

Your curves also give *you* pleasure. Legs, bottoms, thighs, tummies – they're all part of your healthy, functioning, living, breathing body. So think of a slightly dimply bottom as a sign of a rich, happy and fulfilling life.

Oh, and a spongy bottom is also handy at weddings and on bikes; pews and saddles can be so uncomfortable.

So let's start by nipping that self-criticism in the bud. Time, instead, to celebrate that ass. Try some of these today:

✿ Savour the good things about your bum and thighs – that satisfying pain/exhilaration when you cycle up a hill, the sensation of rubbing lovely cream into your legs, someone else fondling your behind...

✿ Every day, promise yourself you'll do something that makes you feel good about your body – have something really delicious to eat, treat yourself to a day at a spa, go for a swim, book a fantastic holiday. Doing something pleasurable can make you feel happy.

✿ Stop buying clothes that don't fit but which you're aiming to 'diet into'. They make you feel worse about your body. Instead, buy yourself something big but gorgeous that you can wear now.

✿ Make a mental list of your best bits – hair, feet, long, beautifully shaped fingernails, trim calves, firm boobs. Stop focusing on your shortcomings and acknowledge your glories.

✿ Splash out on body treats: indulging really does boost your self-confidence – book a facial/manicure, buy new perfume, wallow in a luxurious, gorgeous smelling bath. Take pleasure in looking your best.

✿ Start taking some exercise. It can boost your mood, improve your complexion, help you focus and give you confidence in your body.

Defining idea...

'**Everything has its beauty, but not everyone sees it.**'
CONFUCIUS

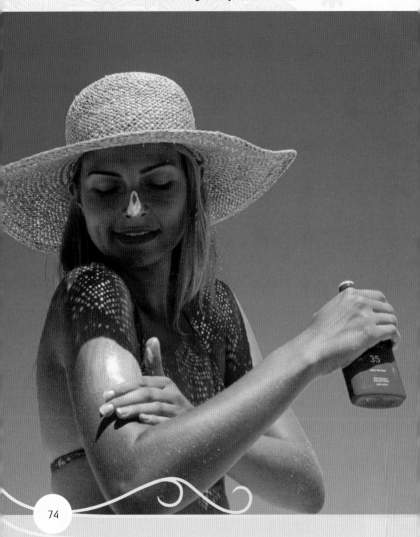

16. Brown girl in the ring

Cellulite looks less obvious on bronzed legs. If you can't beat it...hide it with a fake tan!

Faking it is so much safer than baking in the sun. And many of us would agree that we would be less tempted to soak up the rays if we arrived on holiday with a bit of colour.

It's also brilliant at helping disguise cellulite – fake tan somehow seems to even out those lumps and bumps. Plus the prep work you do before you apply it – exfoliating, moisturising and so on – helps hydrate the area, remove dead skin cells and even out skin-texture. So cellulitey skin can look better already.

Applying fake tan used to be a messy, smelly old business. And the shades were questionable. Mercifully, gone are the days of George Hamilton-style tans in a shade of tangerine that smelt of something you'd keep under the sink.

These days fake tans are sophisticated, easy to use, quick-drying and incredibly effective. They're a great way to prepare your body for your two weeks in the sun, or cover up pasty white bits when you're wearing that sundress/mini-skirt/strappy number. The magic ingredient is DHA (dihydroxyacetene), which turns the skin brown by oxidizing amino acids in the skin. And manufacturers usually add lots of other lovely softening, toning, hydrating ingredients too.

Here's an idea for you...

Fake tanning doesn't have to be a messy, painstaking business. You can buy packets of nifty little self-tan wipes, which you just rub over your skin, and a golden tan appears in a few hours. Keep a packet in your handbag, just in case you need to undress and impress pronto.

Fake tans come in mousses, creams, gels and lotions. Self-applied tans tend to last up to four or five days, or you can go the professional route and visit a specialist, who might put you in a booth and spray you with the stuff. Salon tans tend to last longer – some claim theirs last between a week and a fortnight. A salon is the best route if you want an all-over tan without the hassle of doing it yourself. Best salon choices include St Tropez, Guinot and Clarins.

Here's what to expect if you're a salon tan virgin. You disrobe (and usually pop on a pair of charming paper pants), after which the therapist exfoliates you, and slaps on handfuls of goo, covering you thoroughly. She'll then leave you there for up to an hour while the tanner works its magic, and she then removes the excess. When you shower the next day (if you can leave it that long) you look fantastic. Make sure you wear dark clothes to avoid staining on your clothes. Many fake tans take a few days to look beautifully natural, so if you're preparing for a special do, book your treatment a few days prior to the event.

If you're using a self-tanner at home, make sure you patch test the area beforehand to avoid an allergic reaction. Don't be tempted to go too dark; always choose one that matches your natural skin tone. The best

tried-and-tested self-tanners
include those by Decleor, Ambre
Solaire, St-Tropez and Lancaster.

Follow the three golden rules:
exfoliate, *moisturise* and *layer*.

Defining idea...

'The average man is more interested in a woman who is interested in him than he is in a woman with beautiful legs.'
MARLENE DIETRICH

❀ Start by exfoliating the area with a body scrub, loofah or flannel.
   Apply exfoliator with circular movements (it helps boost circulation).
   paying particular attention to heels, knees and elbows where the
   skin is rougher. A cheaper option is Epsom salts – which will help to
   deep-cleanse your skin. Just fill a cup with salts and add enough
   water to make a paste. Massage over your skin, then rinse off.

❀ Always moisturise after exfoliating. Leave the moisturiser on for
   about fifteen minutes before you apply your fake tan so it doesn't
   interfere with the active ingredient in fake tanning products.

❀ Remove excess moisturiser with a damp flannel before you apply the
   tanning product – especially on bony areas such as knees, elbows and
   ankles – it'll prevent any uneven tanning.

❀ Apply the fake tan, smothering it on as you would a moisturiser.
   Don't forget backs of knees and hands, and your inner thighs.

✿ Then build up gradually. You don't need as much where your skin is thinner as the colour will stay longer here.

✿ Tan usually appears about three or four hours later – if you find you have streaks, try exfoliating the area.

✿ Avoid swimming or having a shower for about twelve hours after a treatment.

✿ Moisturise your body well over the next few days to prolong your fake tan.

✿ And always remember that a fake tan won't protect you from the sun so you still need sunscreen.

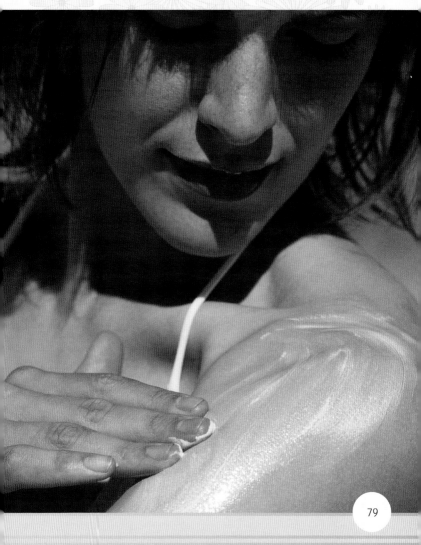

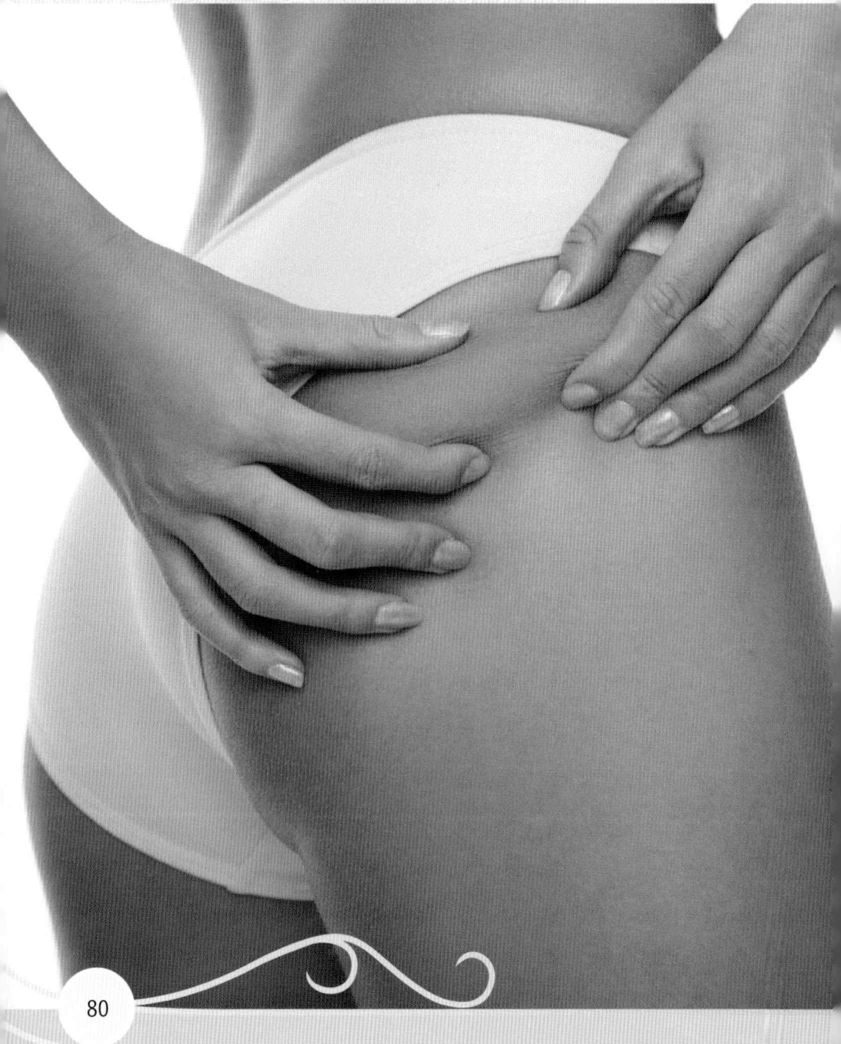

17. On the shelf

Cellulite creams abound. But what works, what doesn't and what's really worth the money?

There's no denying the placebo effect of using cellulite creams – there's nothing like rubbing on pricey, sweet-smelling, beautifully packaged unguents to make you feel you're spoiling yourself.

But, do they work? You might be seduced into thinking so. These days many products are impressively endorsed by various scientific studies, many of which claim that testers lost inches and pounds after using said unguent for a period of time.

But if you're hoping for a miracle in a bottle, you still have a long wait. Cellulite creams alone, however impressive, aren't likely to transform fleshy, saggy buttocks into a nectarine-firm bottom.

But they may certainly help. Cellulite creams can hydrate your skin, so if your thighs and bottom have been neglected, rubbing on a cream will moisturise the area and help plump up the skin. Big difference already.

Many cellulite creams also contain temporary toning ingredients, which help improve skin texture; the effects can be pretty immediate but are temporary – good for a hot date, beach day, black dress occasion, that sort of thing.

Here's an idea for you...

Short on pennies? Try natural olive or grapeseed oil; you can buy them over the counter at chemists for next to nothing. Gentle enough for newborn babies, they're unlikely to cause reactions and are great for massage or for all over moisturising.

But the longer-lasting effects come down to a pot-pourri of active ingredients, which do anything from boost metabolism, facilitate cell turnover, help shed water, even break down fat.

Take *caffeine*, a common and effective ingredient in many anti-cellulite formulations. It's thought to encourage the metabolism of fats, and help drain accumulated fluids in your fat cells, and boost your circulation. It's also toning.

Another key ingredient used in the more effective anti-cellulite creams is *retinol*. It's a derivative of vitamin A that has been found to increase skin renewal and boost the production of collagen. Often found in face cream, it can improve the elasticity of the skin on your nether regions too. RoC's retinol-based product has many devotees, who claim to have lost inches and firmed up significantly using the formulation twice daily.

Another cellulite-busting ingredient is *aminophylline*, which is thought by some experts to enter the bloodstream and actually break down fat in the cells. One study found women using aminophylline cream lost as much as 8 mm from their thighs. Another study showed impressive results with aminophylline, although it was used alongside a calorie-reduced diet and daily exercise too.

Exfoliating ingredients such as *alpha-hydroxy acids* (AHAs) are often used in the latest cellulite-busting products. AHAs are found in plants (citrus fruits and apples) and are used in skin products to help remove dead skin cells, thereby promoting the turnover of new cells. Thus far research has found that the effects on cellulitey areas tend to be temporary, rather than permanent, but watch this space.

Defining idea...

'I will buy any cream, cosmetic, or elixir from a woman with a European accent.'
ERMA BOMBECK, humorist

Natural ingredients

Most treatment creams are a combination of cutting-edge technology alongside tried and trusted natural or herbal ingredients. Here are a few to look out for:

✿ Gingko biloba can stimulate your circulation and boost blood flow. It's a strong antioxidant, so it may help slow down the ageing process and help fight the free radicals that can cause your skin to age.

✿ Gotu kola. This herb is thought to enhance the production of collagen. It's good for circulation and also has diuretic qualities. It's been found to help heal wounds and burns, so has positive effects on skin tissue.

✿ Guarana is a natural stimulant with a strong diuretic action. This seed is thought to help boost metabolism, and also has antioxidant qualities.

✿ Horse chestnut can help reduce water retention, boost circulation and increase blood flow to the skin.

✿ Butcher's broom is a plant extract with a diuretic action and may help boost circulation.

✿ Ivy has been found to help boost the circulation. It also has astringent properties, which may have a temporary toning effect on cellulite.

✿ Marine extracts such as carrageenan and alginic acid can help draw water into the skin, which may help make cellulite look less obvious by filling in the dimples.

✿ Co-enzyme Q10 is a powerful antioxidant thought to help beat cellulite by helping build collagen, thereby countering skin sagginess.

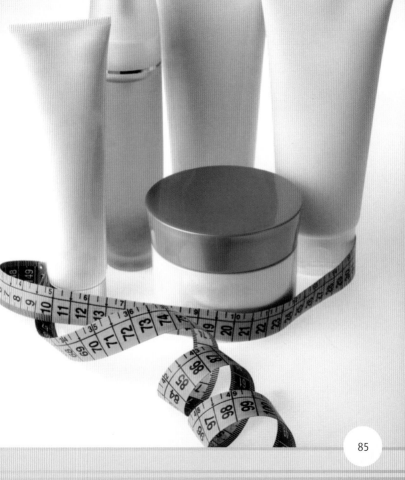

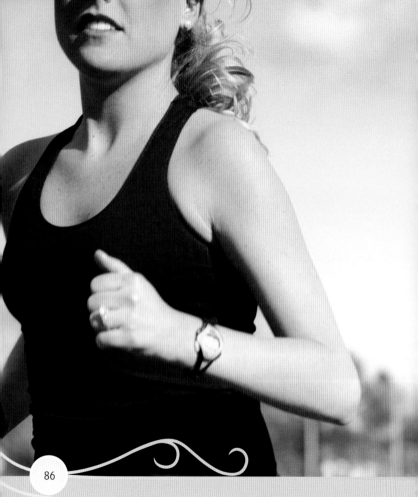

18. Top gear

As you age, your metabolism slows down, which means more body fat, and a saggier bottom and thighs as the years go by. Try some strategies to rev up your body chemistry.

Were you at the back of the queue when they were handing out metabolic rates? 'It's not me, it's my metabolism' is an oft-given excuse for erring on the lardy side.

To a certain extent, your metabolic rate is genetic. Experts say that the rate at which a person burns up calories can vary as much as 25% – that's between people of the same weight.

Your age also affects the rate at which you burn calories. Between the ages of 30 and 80, muscle mass decreases by 40–50%, which reduces your strength and slows down your metabolism.

So, if you've drawn the short straw, and you're gaining weight – and cellulite – as a result, it's time to get tough on your metabolism.

Start by working out how many calories you actually need, based on your metabolic rate. Remember, you gain weight when you take in more calories than you expend.

First, calculate your basal metabolic rate (BMR) – this is the rate at which your body burns energy even when you're not doing anything.

Here's an idea for you...

Drinking 2 litres of still water a day can help your body burn off an extra 150 calories according to one study. It's thought to stimulate the sympathetic nervous system and increase the metabolic rate.

Your BMR = weight in kilos × 2 × 11 (if you prefer to work in pounds that will be your weight in pounds × 11)

So, if you're 65 kilos, your BMR = 65 × 2 × 11 = 1,430.

Now work out how many extra calories you expend according to your lifestyle:

❀ Inactive or sedentary: BMR × 20%.

❀ Fairly active, i.e. you walk and take exercise once or twice a week: BMR × 30%.

❀ Moderately active, i.e. you exercise two or three times a week: BMR × 40%.

❀ Active (you exercise hard more than three times a week): BMR × 50%.

❀ Very active (you exercise hard every day): BMR × 70%.

So if you're a fairly active 65 kg woman, your additional calorie requirement is 1,430 × 30% = 429.

Add this to your BMR to find out how many calories you need a day: 1,430 + 429 = 1,859. So if you eat more than 1,900 calories and don't increase your activity levels, you'll gain weight.

What's the best way to boost your metabolic rate?

Exercise

Move more: incorporate regular aerobic and weight-bearing exercise into your week (running, hill walking or weight training will do). When you increase the amount of lean tissue in your body, you use up more calories even when you're just sitting there; muscle uses more calories than fat does. Aim for 30–40 minute sessions, four or five times a week.

Eat regularly, and don't fast

When you eat less, your metabolism drops because your body tries to conserve energy in case its food supply is about to run out. Small, regular meals are better than scoffing a big meal then eating nothing for hours.

Eat protein

Eating protein uses more calories than other foodstuffs. If you're doing an aerobic workout three to five times a week you need more protein – about 1.1 g of protein for every kilo of body weight. If you're sedentary you need about 0.8 g per kilo of body weight. (As a guide, you get about 44 g of protein in an average lean steak, and about 25 g in a portion of lean chicken.)

Defining idea...

'Genius depends on dry air, on clear skies – that is, on rapid metabolism, on the possibility of drawing again and again on great, even tremendous quantities of strength.'
FRIEDRICH NIETZSCHE

Have a steak occasionally

Red meat and dairy produce contain conjugated linoleic acid (CLA). Research has shown this may increase the amount of lean tissue in your body, which boosts metabolic rate.

Go exotic

Add some chillies to your dishes – apparently they can raise your metabolic rate by about 50% for up to two or three hours after a meal.

Have a pre- and post-exercise nibble

One recent study found that people who performed gentle resistance exercise within two hours of eating a light, carb-based meal boosted their metabolic rate, and burned the food off quicker than those who didn't exercise afterwards. Plus, if you aim to eat something within half an hour of finishing a workout you'll increase your metabolic rate further. After exercising, your body will be low in energy. Replace it quickly and you'll keep your metabolism higher.

Have a coffee break

Caffeine can boost your metabolic rate – partly because it increases your heart rate and also because it makes you fidgety! Don't drink more than two or three cups a day though. Alternatively, try green tea. Studies show that drinking a cup of the green stuff twice daily could help you burn about 70 calories more each day – that's about 3.5 kg in a year! Researchers believe it's the catechins (antioxidants) and other flavonoids in green tea that help boost your metabolism.

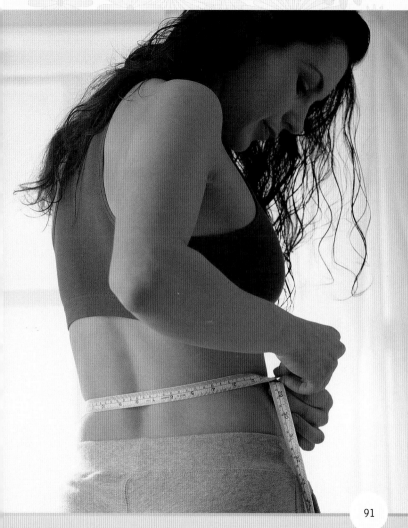

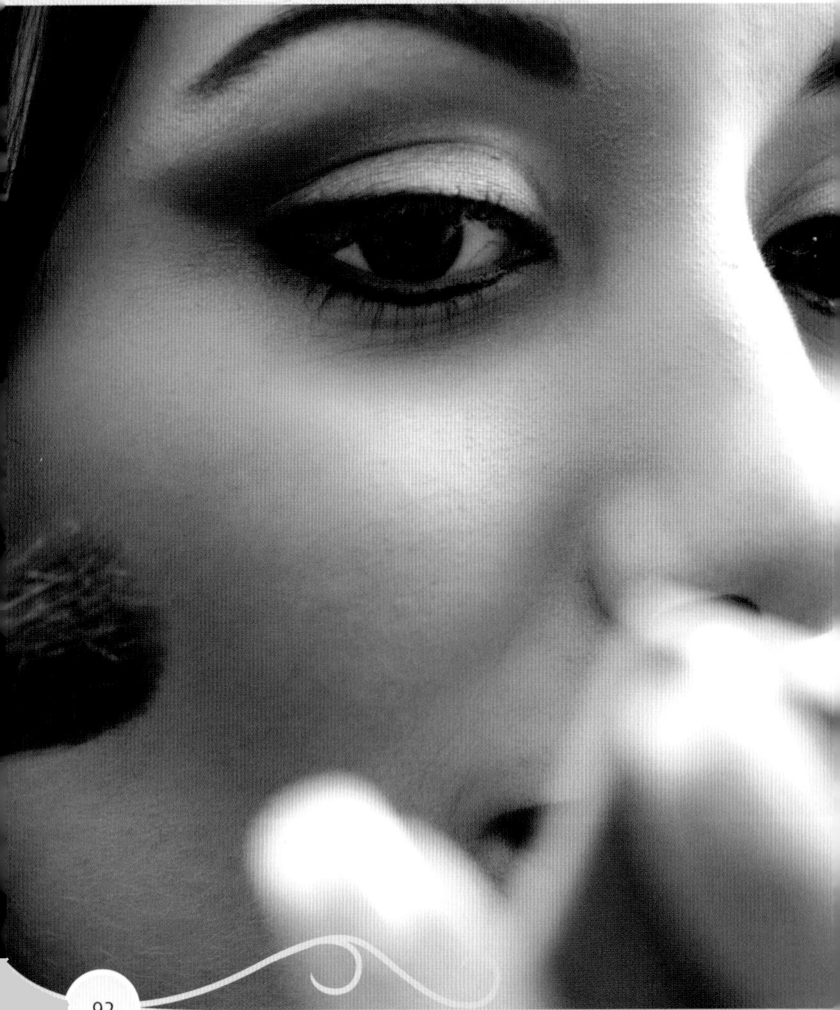

19. Short cuts to supermodel looks

Yes, yes, we know – the key to looking great is lots and lots of sleep, eating well, working out daily, good skin care etc. Surely there must be an easier way.

The problem is that you haven't quite found the time for all that healthy living stuff but what you do have is a date/party/wedding and just a few hours to get ready. To heap up the pressure, you just *have* to shine. It's an emergency. Like your ex is going to be there and you have to make him jealous, even though he's going to be with the current squeeze – who happens to be Angelina Jolie. What to do?

As they said in *Reservoir Dogs*, it's time to go to work. First things first: first impressions do count, so make sure that you have all your necessary maintenance done for your special night out – hair and nails looking great. It's not just the look itself, it's the fact that the psychological boost will leave you with a glow that shows. For a small investment that goes a long way, a manicure is a must.

A full afternoon in the beautician's is the best way to go but if time and money don't permit and you simply have to polish up your crowning glory then the cheat's way to a shiny head of hair is Aveda's Purefume Brilliant Spray On For Hair (www.aveda.com). This adds instant gloss and shine to even the dullest locks.

Here's an idea for you...

Ignore Bridget Jones's nightmare, the gruesome fact is that granny gripper knickers (or 'pants of steel' as India Knight puts it) are the short-term solution to waistline emergencies. On this one, it's only right to go with the advice of India Knight herself (nothing nasty meant by that, India) and get yourself the ultimate pair – Nancy Gantz BodySlimmers High Waist Belly Buster. They are simply the best and the only trick they miss is that they should come complete with a suicide pill on the basis that obviously it is better to die than to let anyone know that they're what you're wearing.

The best way to great skin is a healthy diet and a couple of weeks in fresh air, sea and sun (not forgetting your SPF, natch). However, we're presuming that for you this is just wishful thinking so wipe the McDo remains from your mouth and resort to a facial for short-term cheating. If you can afford the time and the money for a salon-based treat then do so – the more you spend, the better you'll feel. However, if you can't, there's plenty you can do at home. Forget cucumber slices on the eyes – it'll make you feel too much like a distressed divorcee and not enough like a sex kitten. Instead go for the likes of Origins Clear Improvement (www.origins.com), which is a black charcoal mask to draw out pore-clogging impurities, followed by an Elemis Fruit Active Rejuvenating Mask (www.elemis.com).

Remember girls to have a hot bath before you go out to plump out your complexion with all that steam and to get the circulation going so that you appear rosy and, therefore, healthy.

Nutrition is a long-term thing but there are certain short-cutting cheats that will give you an instant hit of feel-good factor. Try taking a slug of supergreens, for instance. Supergreens are ground up superfoods – extremely health promoting vegetables, algae and sprouted grasses – which give a shot of optimum nutrition in one glass. Upside: you'll swear you can actually notice the difference in energy levels and well-being. Downside: they tend to taste disgusting. So, mix these life-giving powders with a little juice and down the hatch. Two that taste just about OK and give you a spring in your step are Kiki's Nature's Living Superfood (www.kiki-health.co.uk) and Perfect Food by Garden of Life (www.gardenoflifeusa.com).

Depending on how fit you are, some people also recommend performing a couple of press ups (yes that's for girls as well as boys) to flush the blood through your system and bring a healthy glow to your skin. Remember, though, healthy glow should not be confused with out of breath and beetroot faced. Before you make your entrance, try spritzing your face with a water spray, which helps cool you down and also freshens up your make up – so carry your own supply with you at all times.

Defining idea...

'Grace in women has more effect than beauty.'
WILLIAM HAZLITT

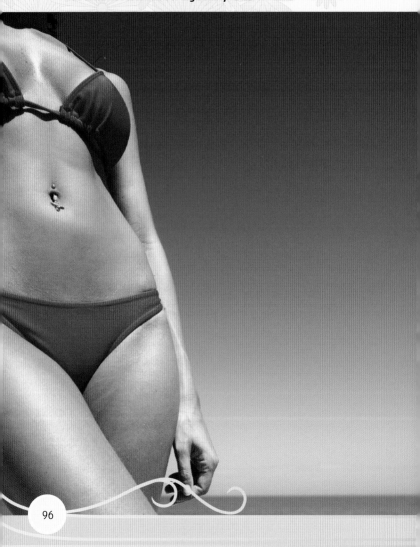

20. Dressing yourself slim

If thinking of a hideously strict diet before that date/interview/holiday drives you to the cake tin, take heart. You can look thinner and more elegant through your choice of clothes.

One of my friends used to be rarely seen out unless in black. Neither did her magazine colleagues. 'It's the media uniform,' she explains, 'the one-colour-suits-all for every event in your working life. And beyond, actually. I'd wear it to every function too – weddings, christenings, bah mitzvahs, garden parties. Even at the kind of outings that begged for the most feminine florals and pastel chiffon, I'd be there head to toe in some billowy – or worse, silhouette-enhancing – black number, believing it made me look barely there thin.'

Black can indeed look supremely elegant – the longer the streak you create, the better. But individual it rarely is. Dark colours certainly can minimise the bulges, but it's not the only sartorial route to a more slender you. Besides it can also be dreary, draining and make you look like 'the help'. Get it ever so slightly wrong at functions and you'll have half a dozen coats flung at you, or be asked for another vol-au-vent, both of which, when you're aiming for willowy Eva Herzigova-esque grandeur, will extinguish the joys of appearing to have a slightly smaller arse.

Here's an idea for you...

Colour experts say white, silver and mother of pearl are 'eternally feminine' because they're associated with the moon, stars and sea. Remember that luminous uber-gown that Nicole Kidman wore to the Oscars ceremony a couple of years ago? If the red carpets invites are thin on the ground for you, invest in striking silver or pearl jewellery instead; it's the easiest way to wear these colours. Alternatively tap into your inner goddess with a soft shell-pink wrap and mother-of-pearl make up – great against a tan. Light colours close to your face can reflect light, and take years off you too.

Instead of black, be inventive. Follow these guidelines:

✿ You can minimise bulges by sticking to one colour – and pretty much any colour. Obviously dark colours are the most flattering, but in summer you can still create the illusion of being longer and leaner if you're dressed head to foot in the same shade, even white.

✿ When you're shopping, make it a rule to ignore size tags. Don't buy the snug size ten just because that's your usual size. You look can lose pounds by wearing slightly looser clothes which skim over bumps and hang flatteringly.

✿ Where possible, choose lined clothes. They won't hug you so unforgivingly. Lined trousers are a godsend, particularly in summer because they drop crisply, however hot and sweaty you are beneath.

❀ Invest in an A line skirt. It flatters almost everyone because it doesn't cling to your curves, and it minimises your bottom. The best length is on, or just below the knee – and if you team it with knee length boots you can disguise thick legs and hefty unfeminine thighs. In the summer a light coloured skirt can look great with suede or denim boots.

Defining idea...

'I have always said that the best clothes are invisible ... they make you notice the person.'
KATHARINE HAMNETT, fashion designer.

❀ Don't be afraid of hipster jeans. They may seem the preserve of nubile girly band members but they can be really flattering whatever your age as they create the illusion of having smaller hips. Just keep a close eye on the flesh overhang because it can ruin the effect. Stick if possible to the boot leg cut – it's even more flattering since it makes your legs look longer and slimmer.

❀ Always wear a heel, however slight. Even tall women can get away with tiny tapering heels. The extra inch or two will add length and can make you more aware of your posture.

❀ Stick to textured fabrics. They can help to 'break up' flesh. Think linen, wool or even crinkled man-made fabrics.

❀ Disguise a big bust with V-necks and low scoop necks. Avoid slash necks and halter necks altogether as they just make you look bulky.

❀ Always choose trousers with hems long enough to skim the tip of a boot or shoe. They may feel too long, but they'll immediately draw the eye down, giving the impression of a longer, leaner leg. And avoid tapered trousers or clam diggers or pedal pushers for the same reason – they make almost everyone's legs look shorter and squatter, and thighs look bigger than they are.

❀ Investing in good lingerie can knock pounds off you; go for well fitting bras with uplift and knickers that flatten in the right places. With bras, aim to banish seams, puckering and surplus flesh bursting out of cups (unless it's what you're aiming for).

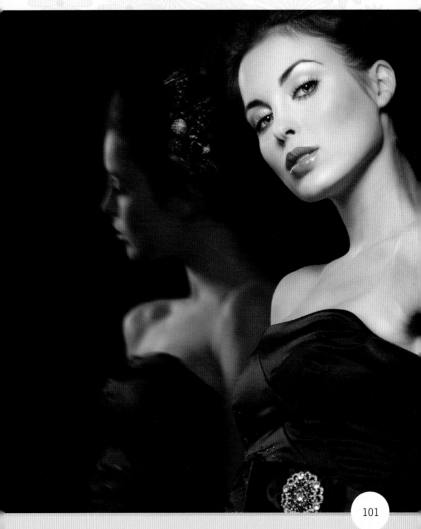

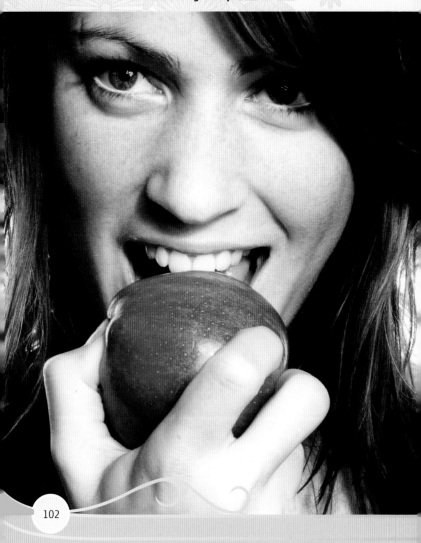

21. It's never too late to change your mind – sticking to a diet

Have you been on diets before, lost weight, then regained it and lost motivation? Change your attitude to dieting and use your mind to get ahead.

I have a friend who's been on every kind of diet going: cabbage soup, high protein, eating for your blood type, meal replacements and all the rest. The trouble is, she hasn't changed her poor mental attitude to dieting.

She uses diets like buses, jumping on and off. If she's just missed one, well, there will be another along in a minute, won't there? Has she lost weight? Yes, she has and then she's gained it, until the next period of dieting when the cycle repeats itself.

Why is it that most diets only seem to work temporarily? In my opinion the main reason is that they don't teach you much about healthy eating or help you learn a healthy attitude to food. All too often, entire food groups are banned, which, depending on the group, can be unhealthy or even dangerous if you follow it for a long time. Meal replacements, although designed nowadays to be nutritionally safe, don't really give the average dieter any idea of what a healthy meal looks like. If a diet promises you rapid weight loss, you can bet it will be due to consuming significantly less calories. It won't be because of some magical fat-

Here's an idea for you...

Drink fruit juice not cola. According to new research from the American Diabetes Association, just one regular can of a fizzy drink a day is enough to increase your risk of diabetes by 85%. A can a day could also lead to a weight gain of around a stone in four years.

burning enzyme found in the bongo-bongo fruit or whatever the angle is! Besides, you'll just lose water and lean muscle mass anyway, so it won't necessarily be sustainable.

Diets can be as dull as ditchwater, particularly if they are very strict about what you can and can't eat. Not only do you feel bored and start fantasising about bathing in jelly and custard (mmm, with some chocolate sprinkles too), but they can make eating out difficult, especially when you visit friends' houses. You have to be very good company indeed to make up for your inconvenient food requests. Let's face it, a diet can simply be hard to fit into your life, particularly when you also have a family to feed or if you work long or unusual hours. And then there's the hunger, the growling stomach and the faintness-inducing pangs that all too often lead to a binge. Then you feel guilty – and move on to another diet in the hope that it will be better.

Many people who sincerely want to lose weight are failing to stick to their diet regimes. So what does work? There isn't one single way to lose weight successfully. You need to develop a combination of tricks that work for you, and an acceptance of certain key points. The first is that you will probably need to change your idea of what a diet and losing weight is all about. The kinds of diets mentioned above are not going to help you. To lose weight and keep it off, you have to change your eating habits and lifestyle permanently. Before you shriek that this sounds even scarier than a wasp-chewing diet, remember that losing weight is about the long haul, not dieting in short four-week bursts. There are no quick fixes, but if you make small changes over a period of time, they will add up to big results.

Defining idea...

'I never worry about diets. The only carrots that interest me are the number you get in a diamond.'
Mae West

Next, you have to realistic about your weight-loss goals. Aim to be in the best shape you can be, which is to be healthy, not to look like a stick insect. Eat a balanced selection of foods with plenty of fruit and vegetables, protein and carbohydrate and a little fat. A balanced diet is essential for good health, keeps things interesting for you and ensures you won't suffer endless cravings because you're denying yourself certain foods. Remember that you do need to keep a check on the portion sizes. You'll also be doing yourself a big favour if you become more physically active. Exercise makes you feel and look good, helps to control your appetite and, in conjunction with sensible eating, helps you lose weight faster. Using these guidelines, weight should come off slowly but surely, without you feeling as though you've put your entire life on hold to accommodate a short-term diet. You might just enjoy yourself too!

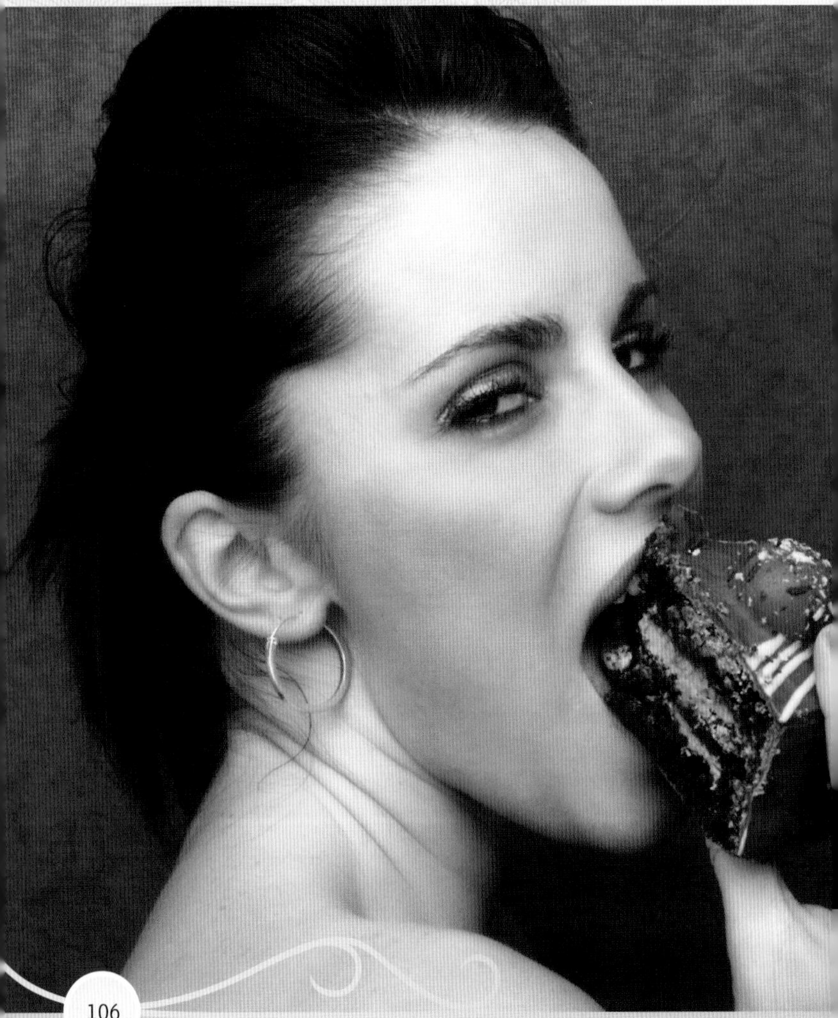

22. Are you an emotional eater?

If you find that you often eat without being truly hungry, perhaps it's time to work out what's eating you instead.

On a physical level food is simply fuel for the body, yet our relationship with it is complex. It is a story filled with love and hate.

We read books about food, watch TV programmes about it and pay lots of money to go and eat what someone else cooks for us at restaurants. Over the years we learn habits and behaviours around food that can become inappropriate. These are often rooted in well-meaning parenting. How many of us polish off every last morsel from our plates because mum told us that the poor kids in Africa are starving or that in her generation all they got was bread, potatoes and water? How many of us will have a sweet treat in response to physical or emotional pain, recalling being soothed with confectionery after a childhood fall? We even give foods a moral value – some are bad or sinful, while others are good and virtuous.

It's a rollercoaster of a relationship, which is fine if you don't have any issues with weight. If you do, and food seems to be controlling you, remember you are not alone. Thousands of us are stuck in this kind of one-way relationship. You need to work out why you are feeding your emotions and what you will do about it.

Here's an idea for you...

Eat more slowly. It takes 20 minutes for 'I'm full' signals to reach the brain. Work with your body by giving it the time it needs to respond.

The desire to eat is masterminded in the brain and involves more than twenty different chemical messengers in your body. Eating anything will stave off hunger, but not overwhelming cravings for a particular type of food. If you are hungry you have to eat, but when you want to eat for any other reason, you need to develop coping strategies that don't involve food. It is usually the negative emotions that drive us to munch more – unhappiness, stress and boredom, for instance. Different approaches work for different people; coping tactics could include talking to a friend, doing some physical exercise, confronting a situation at work that is troubling you or scheduling in some 'me time', such as a fun shopping trip, a facial or a game of golf. The point is to identify the where, when and how of your emotionally reactive eating and deal with that rather than continuing the behaviour that's holding your diet to ransom.

Another trigger can be tiredness. Again, you need to get to the root cause. Are you exhausted because of work pressure or certain relationships? Or is it because night after night you go to bed too late? Tiredness lowers your mood, which makes you want to eat and perk yourself up, and it also makes your body send hunger signals because it is looking for more energy to get you through the day.

My downfall is boredom and procrastination. I often look for the answers to life in the fridge. I can also spend a long time seeking inspiration in a slice of cheesecake, especially the lovely crunchy bit at the bottom. The cure is to do something more interesting than the thing you're putting off. Alternatively, set yourself mini goals; for example, if you finish a task in one hour you will then reward yourself (not with food) before tackling the next task.

Defining idea...

'Stressed spelled backwards is desserts. Coincidence? I don't think so.'
ANONYMOUS

You don't have to finish up everything on your plate. You could try ordering or cooking a smaller portion to begin with. If you need to assuage guilty feelings, pledge some money to charity for every kilo of weight you lose.

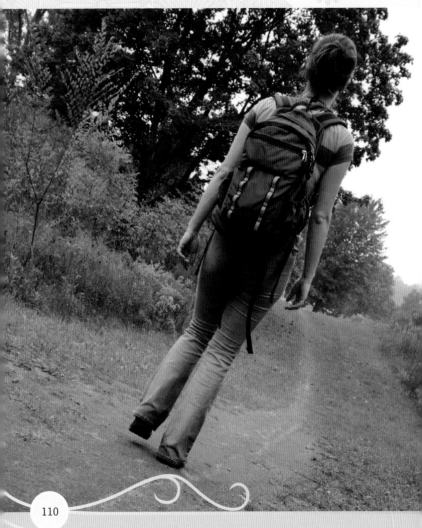

23. Walk yourself thinner

If you're new to exercise or just don't fancy the gym, here's a simple way to drop some weight. It's easy to start, and requires no special clothing or equipment.

Most of us view walking as a way to get from A to B, and most of the time we'll choose to use the car or bus to get us to where we want to go.

There is a good reason to put one foot in front of the other more often: it's a great way to lose weight and stay slim. It is not expensive, it is not complicated and you can do it anywhere.

Half an hour's walking will burn up an average of about two hundred calories and help to tone up your legs and bottom. There's a catch; you won't see results with a gentle stroll to work or the shops once or twice a week. To make a difference, you'll need to walk at least three times a week, building up to five times a week, for half an hour. You'll need to do it at a reasonable pace, one that warms you up, makes you feel ever so slightly sweaty and leaves you feeling slightly breathless, but not so breathless that you could not hold a conversation. If you walk up some hills or on an incline on the treadmill in the gym, you'll increase the challenge and burn up more calories. It is simple. Here are a few other pointers to bear in mind:

Here's an idea for you...

Make your dairy product intake low-fat. In research, obese volunteers lost 11% of their body weight over six months on a calorie-controlled diet that included three low-fat dairy portions a day.

✿ You don't really need specialist gear for walking, but a decent pair of trainers will support you better than ordinary shoes. If you're planning to take up hill walking or hiking, you will need shoes or boots designed for the purpose, both for comfort and safety.

✿ You'll work harder outdoors than inside on a treadmill as you'll have to cope with changing terrain and wind resistance. This is a good thing as you'll burn calories faster and get extra toning benefits. Regularly spending time outside has been shown to keep you emotionally fit too, boosting feelings of well-being and staving off depression.

✿ Wear something comfortable! It might sound obvious, but if you get wet or too hot, you'll want to give up and go back home. High-tech sports fabrics are designed to draw away sweat and protect you from wind and rain without weighing you down.

✿ When walking, keep your tummy muscles pulled in to work your abdominal muscles and protect your back. Walk tall, avoid slumping and use your natural stride.

✿ If you swing your arms while you walk, you'll increase your heart rate and get more of a workout.

Defining idea...

'Walking is the best possible exercise.'
Thomas Jefferson

✿ For the best technique, hit the ground with your heel first, roll through your foot and then push off with your toes.

Rather than just randomly walking when you feel like it, try to schedule a daily walk, or at least every other day. That way, you are more likely to stick with it and see results in conjunction with your healthier eating habits, plus you'll be able to monitor your progress.

To reap the greatest benefits, set yourself a plan, say over six weeks, gradually increasing the length of time you walk and its frequency and the speed. For example, in week one you could walk for half an hour three times a week, slowly for 15 minutes and briskly for 15 minutes. Over the next few weeks, you would aim to add another walking session and making each one 5 or 10 minutes longer, and you would walk briskly for 20 or 25 minutes and at a slower pace for the rest of the time. By the end of six weeks, you could be walking for 45 minutes to an hour four or five times a week, and mostly at the faster pace. You'll be seeing a slimmer you in the mirror.

Defining idea...

'A sedentary life is the real sin against the Holy Spirit. Only those thoughts that come by walking have any value.'
Friedrich Nietzsche

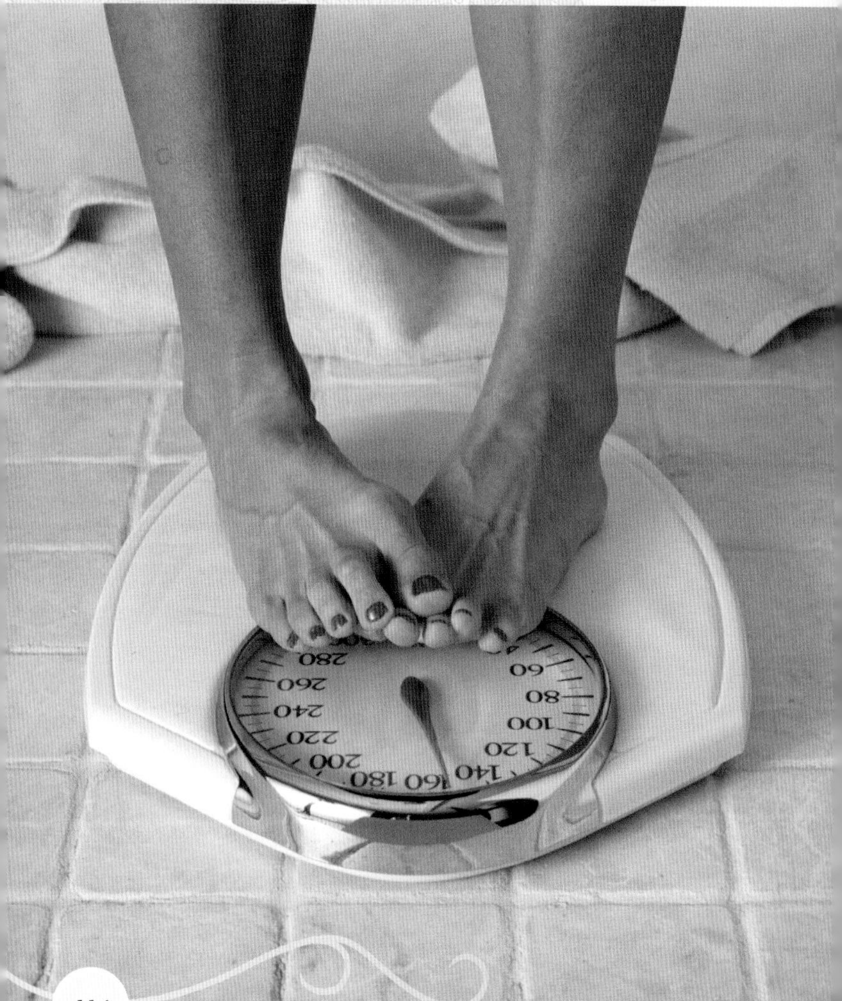

24. Stuck on those last 7lbs?

That stubborn half a stone is hard to shift whether you are near the end of your weight loss programme or when 7 lb is all you want to lose to begin with.

It's such a small amount, you'd think it would pack its bags and leave without a whimper. But no, that half a stone always seems to be trickiest to shift.

I don't know why, but what I do know is that to make it go away you have to re-double your efforts and have more tricks up your sleeve than a magician. Make a start with my ten-point checklist.

1.   Be honest with yourself about what you're eating. Keep a food diary for a week and note down everything that you consume. You might think you're eating sensibly, but a diary could help you spot the source of those extra kilos.

2.   Do you suffer from portion distortion? Even healthy diet-friendly foods such as fruits have calories. If you eat vast amounts of anything and it exceeds your calorie output, you'll put on weight. Match it and you'll maintain that extra half stone.

3.   How consistent are you? There are some experts who say as long as you eat sensibly for 80% of the time, you can relax a little for the other 20%. This could translate as making the healthiest choices all week and then eating whatever you like at the weekend. However, there's a big

Here's an idea for you...

Limit your food options:
too many choices can make you eat more.
Research has shown that volunteers ate 44%
more than a control group when offered a
variety of dishes rather than the same
amount of one dish.

difference between relaxing a little and having a total blow-out every weekend. If you opt for the blow-outs, your week's calorie intake will stack up and your healthful efforts will be for nothing. That dull word 'moderation' springs to mind, but it really is a good concept to live by.

4. Be more active, whatever your current levels of activity, to rev up your rate of weight loss. If you are sedentary start walking or swimming, ideally for at least half an hour five times a week. They are both safe effective exercises that, if done regularly, will pay dividends. If you are reasonably active, or even if you think you work out a lot, try to incorporate some new activities into your week to challenge your mind and body. Try working out for longer, more frequently or harder – or all of these together!

5. A simple way to cut a few calories is to cut out carbohydrates with your evening meal. You could try it every night for a couple of weeks, or every other night if that's more convenient. As long as your other meals and snacks are nutrionally balanced with some carbohydrate, you won't be missing out and you'll definitely see a difference of the scales.

6. Have healthy snacks. If you eat regular well-balanced meals and have a few in-between snacks that are also healthy – not a packet

of crisps or bar of chocolate –
your blood sugar levels will
remain stable and you won't
ever feel ravenously hungry,
so you're less likely to binge
or overeat.

Defining idea...

**'It's OK to let yourself go, just as long as
you let yourself back.'**
Mick Jagger

7.   Spice up your life with a few hot peppers in your lunch or dinner.
     Pepper eaters have less of an appetite and feel full quicker according
     to Canadian research. The compound capsaicin that is found in
     peppers temporarily speeds your metabolism.

8.   Include calcium in your diet, as, along with other substances in dairy
     foods, it seems to help your body burn excess fat faster. In a study,
     women who ate low fat yoghurt and cheese and drank low fat milk
     three or four times in a day lost 70% more body fat than women
     who didn't eat dairy at all.

9.   Get your rest. Sleep deprivation and a stressed out lifestyle can boost
     levels of cortisol in your body, which is associated with higher levels
     of insulin and fat storage. We can interpret the body's cues for sleep
     as hunger and end up snacking or drinking gallons of coffee to stay
     awake…and then not be able to sleep.

10. Don't eat when you're not hungry. It seems obvious, but think
     about it next time you put your food in your mouth. Ask yourself
     "Am I really hungry?" before that second mouthful.

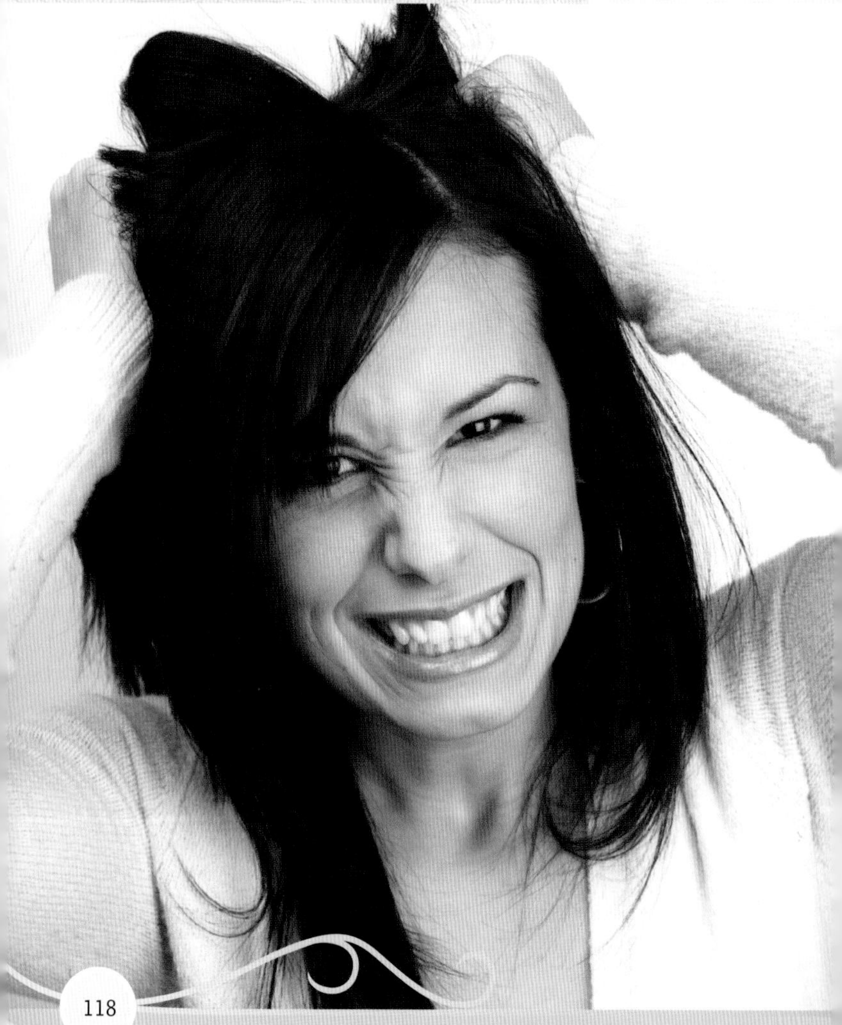

25. Is stress making you fat?

Any sort of stress can lead to weight gain.

Stress causes your body to release cortisol and this stimulates the fat-storing hormone, insulin. Insulin causes your body to hold on to its fat stores.

And that's if you're eating what you always ate. The trouble is that you might be sabotaging yourself without realising it. When we're stressed there's a tendency to overeat, especially carbohydrates. (It's not called comfort food for nothing.) That's because carbohydrates cause the brain to release serotonin and this is one of the feel-good hormones that raise mood. In a way, it's a form of self-medication.

As is booze. Terrific at relaxing you. Fabulous for adding layers of fat around your waistline.

Stay svelte even when stressed
It's not what you eat it's when you eat it

Researchers discovered that when women ate 'off piste' – whenever they wanted – they ate 120 calories a day more than those women who ate three meals and three snacks a day at set times. Decide on your meal times and stick to them. No grazing.

Here's an idea for you...

When you're stressed and feel the temptation to reach for comfort food, try sucking on half a teaspoon of honey instead (manuka honey from New Zealand is especially beneficial). Honey causes the brain to release the feel-good hormone serotonin almost immediately. You might find that just that tiny amount will satisfy you and prevent you pigging out on a bar of chocolate or a packet of biscuits which also cause serotonin release but pack a lot more calories.

Make a conscious effort to cut out salt

We can feel more drawn to salty foods when we're stressed. There could be a physiological reason for this. Salt raises blood pressure and that in turn actually raises cortisol levels – which might have been an advantage when we only got stressed once a month but is redundant for the most part now. Wean yourself from adding salt to food and aim to eat no more than 6 g of salt a day in processed food. If the levels are given in sodium then multiply by 2.5 to get the grams of salt.

Get into green tea

Caffeine raises levels of stress hormones and makes you even more stressed. Try green tea. It has about half the caffeine of coffee and a little less than black tea. And it's good for your brain and your circulation as well as your waistline. There's another advantage. A recent Japanese study found that people drinking green tea lost 2.4 kg (5.3 lb) after 3 months, while those who drank black tea lost only 1.3 kg (2.9 lb). It's also thought that chemicals called catechins found in green tea trigger weight loss.

Savour food

Apparently, it takes 20 minutes for our stomach to register that we've started to eat and switch off the feeling of hunger. It's certainly borne out by a small US study of women who were instructed to eat slowly, chewing each mouthful carefully, savouring their food. These women were told to stop eating when their most recent bite didn't taste as good as the first. They lost 3.6 kg (8 lb). In the same period of time, the control group gained 1.3 kg (3 lb). Our bodies know when we've had enough if we slow down long enough to listen.

Relax

One study showed that women who made a conscious effort to relax lost an average of 4.5 kg (10 lb) in 18 months without consciously dieting. The truth is you need actively to relax in order to switch off the stress hormones which could be contributing to weight gain.

Compete with yourself

The best possible antidote to stress *and* weight gain is to exercise. Buy a pedometer from a sports shop. Measure how many steps you take in an average day (most people average around 4,000), and then do a few more steps each day until you reach 10,000.

Defining idea...

'My doctor told me to stop having intimate dinners for four, unless there are three other people.'
ORSON WELLES